# *How to Sleep Like a Baby,*
## *Wake Up Refreshed, and Get More Out of Life*

Also by Dianne Hales

THE U.S. ARMY TOTAL FITNESS PROGRAM
(with Lt. Col. Robert E. Hales, M.D.)

THE COMPLETE BOOK OF SLEEP

NEW HOPE FOR PROBLEM PREGNANCIES

AN INVITATION TO HEALTH
(3 editions)

# How to Sleep Like a Baby, Wake Up Refreshed, and Get More Out of Life

## DIANNE HALES

Ballantine Books • New York

For Bob and Julia,
who light up the days and the nights of my life,
with love.

Library of Congress Catalog Card Number: 86-91573

ISBN: 0-345-33825-1

Cover design by Richard Aquan
Photo: © Jan Cobb/The Image Bank
Manufactured in the United States of America

First Edition: May 1987

10  9  8  7  6  5  4  3  2  1

# Contents

# How to Sleep Like a Baby,
## Wake Up Refreshed, and Get More Out of Life

# Introduction

Several years ago, when I spoke on sleep to an international group of editors in Switzerland, I was introduced as a *Schlaffschrifter*—a sleepwriter. The description fits, for I've written two books and more than two dozen articles on sleep.

I did my first sleep story back in 1974. At a hospital laboratory in New York City, I watched as researchers attached tiny electrodes to the faces and scalps of volunteers who slept for science's sake. Elaborate monitoring devices translated their brain waves, heart beats, eye movements, and muscle activity into wavy rhythms. To me, the squiggles of data from their sleeping brains and bodies were as mysterious as an undecipherable hieroglyphic. But the men and women at the monitoring machines had cracked the code. They were as excited as astronauts exploring an uncharted new world.

I've come to share their fascination because I've realized

that sleep is more than just a "story." Over the years that I've worked as a medical writer, I've found that whatever the topic, many of my assignments have ended up somehow connected to sleep.

When I wrote about aging, I learned that no other behavior changes as much in the course of a lifetime as our sleep patterns. When I did stories on stress, I realized that sleep enhances our ability to cope with change and challenge. When I reported on mental illness, I saw that troubled sleep sometimes reflects a troubled mind.

When I wrote about the sexes, I found out that a man and a woman sharing the same name, the same life-style, the same house, even the same bed could be worlds apart in their sleep styles. When I did books on fitness, I learned that a good night's sleep is absolutely essential for stamina and strength.

In reporting on health, I've also seen Americans make many healthful changes in the way we live. We spend millions of dollars each year on natural foods, aerobics classes, exercise tapes, workout equipment, diet guides. Yet many people still ignore one crucial aspect of well-being: the third of our lives that we spend asleep.

Unfortunately, millions of us—perhaps as many as one out of every three—cannot sleep as well as we'd like. Many, wide-eyed and desperate, lie in bed for hours before falling asleep. Others wake in the lonely hours after midnight and cannot return to rest. Some barely manage to pull themselves out of bed in the morning. Hundreds of thousands yawn through the afternoon, not realizing that their drowsiness is related to their nighttime rest—or, more precisely, restlessness.

I've written this book for these "walking weary." While a few sleep disorders can be diagnosed and treated only by specialists in sleep medicine, you can tackle the most common sleep difficulties on your own. This book will show you how. I hope that it helps you to sleep better by night and feel better by day, to get the rest of your life—and the best out of life.

# CHAPTER 1

# A Bedtime Story: What Goes On When the Lights Go Out

*I*t's time for bed. Your eyelids droop. Your limbs grow heavy. Stretching and sighing, you climb between the sheets and turn out the light. But you can't turn off your racing mind or restless body. You toss. You turn. You yawn. You yearn. In the blackness of the night, you worry: You aren't going to be able to sleep—not now when you're drowsy, not later when you're desperate, maybe not ever again.

You're hardly alone in your midnight misery. Researchers estimate that 100 million Americans have occasional or chronic problems sleeping. As one wit observed, "If sleep knits up the raveled sleeve of care, a sizable segment of the population is coming a bit unwound." Sleep disorders may plague more men and women than the all-too-common cold.

But while you have to suffer through a cold, you don't have to resign yourself to nights without rest and days without zest. You *can* sleep better by night and feel better by day. Without pills. Without expensive and extensive tests. Without treatments that make you more miserable than insomnia ever did. In fact, you can do more to improve your sleep than anyone or anything else. This book will show you how. But before you begin sleeping better, you have to understand more about sleep itself.

## NIGHT LIFE

Although you may not realize it, you live two lives—one in the waking world and one behind closed lids. In all, you spend a third of your life asleep, or more than 220,000 hours over the course of seventy years. You may think that during this time your sleeping body is like a car parked for the night: motionless, engine off, headlights dimmed. It is anything but.

During sleep, muscles tense and relax. Pulse, temperature, and blood pressure rise and fall. Chemicals crucial for well-being course through the bloodstream. The brain, like a Hollywood producer, conjures up fantastic stories, complete with cliff-hanger plots and dazzling special effects. In fact, so much happens during sleep that it's astounding that we manage to sleep at all.

To understand the process of sleep, imagine yourself descending a staircase. As you close your eyes and drift off, you take a small step down into the first stage of what is called quiet sleep. Stage 1 is a sort of twilight zone between waking and sleep. If roused, you'd probably jerk awake quickly and deny that you'd slept at all. If you were hooked up to an EEG (electroencephalogram), your brain would produce irregular, rapid electrical waves. Your muscle tension decreases. You breathe smoothly, and mundane thoughts float through your mind.

The next step takes you down into stage 2 of quiet sleep.

1. EEG (brain wave record) Awake.

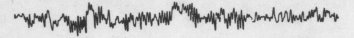

2. EEG Stage 2 Sleep. Brain waves are characterized by sudden bursts of activity.

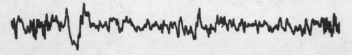

3. EEG Stage 4 Sleep. In this most profound state of unconsciousness, very large brain waves appear in a slow, jagged pattern.

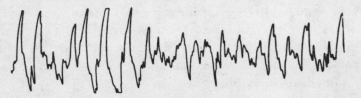

4. EEG REM or "Active" Sleep. Brain waves are pinched and irregular, resembling the patterns of waking more than deep sleep.

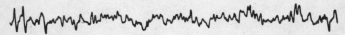

Adapted from *A Primer on Sleep and Dreaming* © 1978 by Rosalind D. Cartwright.

Your brain waves become larger, punctuated by occasional sudden bursts of electrical activity. You've definitely crossed the border between wakefulness and sleep. If someone lifted your eyelids gently, you wouldn't waken; your eyes no longer respond to stimuli.

As you descend into stage 3, your brain waves become slower and bigger. In this state of deep slumber, your bodily functions slow down even more. Finally, stepping down into stage 4, you reach deepest sleep, the most

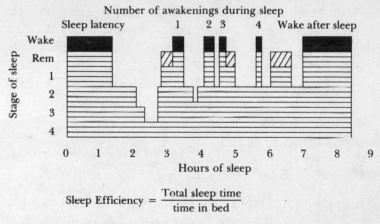

A typical all-night sleep pattern. Courtesy Milton Kramer, M.D., Bethesda Oaks Hospital, Cincinnati, Ohio.

profound state of unconsciousness. On an EEG, your brain waves would appear extremely large and slow. You are so "dead to the world" that even a thunderstorm might not waken you.

This step-by-step journey into oblivion usually takes more than an hour. Then you begin to climb upward, moving rapidly through the same sleep stages as before, not all the way to full wakefulness but into active sleep. Because the pupils dart back and forth, this stage is called Rapid Eye Movement or REM sleep. (The four stages of quiet sleep are often referred to as non-REM or NREM sleep.)

During REM, your brain waves resemble those of waking rather than of quiet sleep. The large muscles of your torso, arms, and legs are paralyzed, although your fingers and toes may twitch. You breathe quickly and shallowly; the flow of blood through your brain accelerates. REM sleep is the time of vivid dreaming, and if wakened, you'd probably recall a tantalizing fragment of a fantasy.

After about ten minutes in REM sleep, you descend the sleep staircase again. The entire cycle of REM and NREM stages takes roughly ninety minutes. Early in the night, the periods spent in the deepest stages of quiet sleep are longer. In the second half of the night, REM sleep predominates. By morning, you go around the sleep circuit four or five times.

## THE NIGHTS OF YOUR LIFE

Throughout a lifetime, no physiological process changes more than sleep needs and patterns. A newborn may spend up to eighteen hours asleep. By age ten, a child requires only nine or ten hours. The best sleepers of all are preteens. They fall asleep within five or ten minutes, sleep for nine and a half hours, and spend 95 percent of their time in bed in solid, continuous, deep sleep—the best rest of a lifetime. By adulthood, seven or eight hours usually provide adequate rest; in old age, six may suffice.

More than total sleep time changes with age, however. The passing years affect the quality as well as the quantity of our sleep. From infancy to adulthood, as total sleep time decreases by more than half, REM periods dwindle to less than a quarter of a night's sleep. By their thirties, men sleep somewhat less deeply; women begin getting less deep sleep in their fifties. By age sixty-five, the proportion of time both sexes spend in deep sleep is half that at age twenty-five. Both stages 1 and 2—the lighter sleep stages—increase. REM shrinks to about a fifth of total sleep time.

In old age, sleep often becomes more fragmented, and the number of nighttime arousals has more of an impact on daytime alertness than the actual hours of sleep—even if the wakenings are so brief they aren't remembered. In a seven-hour sleep period, a healthy senior citizen averages

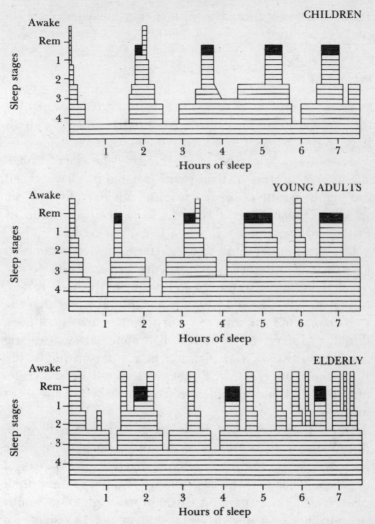

An idealized night's sleep in children, normal young adults, and the elderly. Adapted from A. Kales, "Sleep and Dreams: Recent Research on Clinical Aspects," *Annals of Internal Medicine* 68 (May 1968): 1081.

153 arousals. By comparison, a twenty-five-year-old wakens only ten times.

## WHY SLEEP?

Whatever your age or sleep stage, you ultimately sleep for the same reason: You must. Although some individuals have gone days without rest, sooner or later they succumbed to sleepiness. No other force may be as irresistible. Yet after centuries of living with what some have called the gentle tyrant of sleep, no one can explain why we spend so much time at rest. In fact, sleep, the basis of myths and mysteries, remains a biological riddle.

Unable to understand sleep, different societies came up with their own theories for this curious state. The people of Fiji thought the soul went wandering as the body rested, so they never wakened sleepers abruptly for fear that the soul might not have time to return. Some ancient cultures, thinking of sleep as an intermediate state between waking and death, feared it as a time when a person might slip from night into eternity. Others considered sleep a realm of deities and built temples in which to worship the lords of the night.

Some anthropologists have suggested that nature induced sleep to keep early man out of harm's way. The human race might never have survived the perils of darkness if sleep hadn't kept the first families safe in their caves rather than roaming through the night. But in our neon-lit, nonstop world, we no longer need to sleep for safety's sake. Does that mean that sleep has become an anachronism?

Sleep researcher Allan Rechtschaffen of the University of Chicago thinks not: "If sleep doesn't serve an absolutely vital function, then it's the biggest mistake the evolutionary process ever made. How could sleep have remained virtually unchanged as a monstrously useless, maladaptive vestige throughout the whole of mammalian evolution while selection has, during the same period of time, been able to achieve all kinds of finely tuned adjustments in the shape of fingers and toes?"

Yet no one knows exactly what makes sleep so important. Aristotle associated it with a cooling of the vapors of the head. Shakespeare described it as the "balm of hurt minds, great nature's second course; chief nourisher in life's feast." Freud saw it as a symbolic journey back to the security of the womb. Pavlov thought of it as a conditioned response.

Modern scientists have contended that sleep repairs the ravages of the day, purges our brains of extraneous information, conserves energy, allows time for body maintenance. Perhaps none of these theories is correct; perhaps they all are. Sleep, like waking, may fulfill not just one primary need but many.


## HOW MUCH SLEEP IS ENOUGH?

"Nature requireth five hours' sleep; custom taketh seven; idleness takes nine; and wickedness eleven," states one English proverb. Another gives a different prescription: "Six hours' sleep for a man, seven for a woman, and eight for a fool."

Despite such folklore, there is no one formula for how long a good night's sleep should be. For some people, six hours may be too long to loll in bed; for others, eight might not be enough. Expecting all people to sleep for the same amount of time is as absurd as expecting them to wear the same size shoes.

The range of normal sleep times is from five to ten hours; the average is seven and one-half hours. About one or two people in a hundred can get by with just five; another small minority needs twice that amount. But each individual seems to have an innate sleep "appetite" that's as much a part of genetic programming as hair color, height, and skin tone.

A simple way to figure out your sleep needs is to get up at the same time every morning, regardless of when you go to bed. Are you groggy after six hours of shut-eye? Does an extra hour give you more energy? What about two more hours? Since too much time in bed can make you feel sleepier, you may find that more sacktime isn't necessarily better. Listen to your body's signals, and adjust your sleep habits to suit them.

You may discover that you're a naturally short sleeper, like Napoleon, Thomas Edison, Frederick the Great, Virgil, Horace, Darwin, and George Bernard Shaw, and require only two or three hours of rest a night. Edison, who hated any wastage of time, once commented that "most people overeat 100 percent and oversleep 100 percent." Yet Einstein regularly slept ten hours or more and credited many of his ideas to his long rests.

What's most remarkable about short sleepers is not how little they sleep but how well. They spend just as much time in the deep-sleep stages as longer sleepers but much less time in the lighter "filler" stages of non-REM sleep. Long sleepers rest more lightly, wake more often, and often feel less refreshed in the morning than short sleepers.

In his studies of sleepers, psychiatrist Ernest Hartmann of Boston found intriguing daytime differences between big sleepers, who averaged eight and one-half hours in bed, and little sleepers, who logged a mere five and one-half hours. As he described them, the short sleepers were "efficient, energetic, ambitious persons who tended to work hard and keep busy . . . definitely not worriers; they seldom left themselves time to sit down and think about problems."

The long sleepers were a different breed: "not very sure

of themselves, their career choices or their life-styles; however, several were artistic or creative. . . . [They seemed to be] constantly 'reprogramming' themselves as opposed to the relatively 'preprogrammed' short sleepers."

## DOING WITHOUT

Even though a good night's sleep is the foundation of good daytime health, we can function with less rest than we'd like. In fact, we can get by without any sleep at all— temporarily. In 1959 radio disc jockey Peter Tripp stayed awake without interruption for two hundred hours as part of a fund-raising marathon. He appeared unaffected until the final days, when he began imagining that he heard sounds that didn't exist and that unknown enemies were after him. He became so suspicious of others that he refused to cooperate on performance tests.

In 1964 Randy Gardner, a seventeen-year-old high school student in San Diego, decided to set a record for wakefulness as a science project. Young, healthy, and motivated, Randy stayed awake for eleven days and, while he did become tired, he didn't develop any bizarre behaviors. He held a press conference before going to bed and, after nearly fifteen hours of slumber, resumed his normal sleep-wake patterns.

Chances are that Peter Tripp, Randy Gardner, and other "sleep resisters" actually did rest for periods so brief they're called micro-sleeps. These tiny time-outs may have saved their lives. When laboratory rats were forced to remain awake in order to keep walking and avoid falling into a pool of water, they weakened and died within days. Identical rats, subjected to the same stress but allowed to sleep briefly, survived with few ill effects. "This is a new and important finding about sleep," says Stephen Kennedy, Ph.D., a sleep researcher at the National Institute of Mental Health. "Quite simply, without it, we die."

But even when sleeplessness isn't total or fatal, it can take an enormous toll on mind and body. In a study of sleep-deprived medical residents at William Beaumont Army Medical Center in El Paso, acute sleep loss clearly impaired the young doctors' ability to perform complex mental tasks, sapped their energy levels, made them more depressed and irritable, and triggered inappropriate emotional reactions.

Sleepy people have to struggle so hard just to remain awake that they can't possibly function at their physical or mental peaks. Yet sleepiness has become a nationwide epidemic. In a survey of sleep disorders centers, daytime tiredness was the number-one complaint of those seeking help. According to recent estimates, about 15 percent of the population may be yawning throughout the day.

## SUNRISE, SUNSET

Ecclesiastes recognized an essential truth about life: It has rhythm. To every purpose under heaven, there is indeed a time and a season. More babies are born at 4:00 A.M. than at any other time of day; more people die of disease between 6:00 and 8:00 A.M. than in any other period. Yet of all the rhythms of daily life, none is more significant than our sleep-wake cycle.

Nature seems to have designed this rhythm for a 25-hour day. Cut off from all time cues, volunteers naturally extend their day by about an hour, going to bed later at night and rising later the next morning. Blind individuals, unable to respond to light and darkness, tend to live by a daily cycle of 24.9 hours. Yet most of us learn to live comfortably within the 24 hours of the conventional day. We keep our biological clocks ticking in harmony with man-made ones with the help of time cues or *zeitgebers*.

One of the most powerful is body temperature. Usually we heat up gradually during the day, with our temperatures peaking at midafternoon and bottoming out between midnight and 3:00 or 4:00 A.M. The higher your temperature, the more wide-awake you are, and the better you feel and function.

The best time for bed is when your temperature is dropping: You fall asleep sooner and sleep longer. If you stay up too long, perhaps because of travel or work, and your temperature starts to climb, your total sleep time will decrease. In one experiment where volunteers postponed their bedtime from 11:00 P.M. to 11:00 A.M., they slept 3.5 hours less, even though they'd been awake sixteen to twenty-eight hours longer than usual.

Light also shapes the rhythms of our days and nights. In animals, pulses of light can either delay or advance rest periods. In humans, exposure to light in the morning advances some people's sleep cycles—starting earlier in the day—while light in the evening delays them. No one knows exactly how light resets our biological clocks, but we have proof that it does: By exposing men and women to bright light at different times, scientists have induced changes in blood levels of melatonin, a hormone normally released by the pineal gland only during the night.

Other external factors also affect internal timing: the length of day or night, mealtimes, food, stimulants such as caffeine. One of the strongest time cues seems to be the rhythm of other humans. A baby, born without any sense of night and day, sleeps erratically until it begins to mimic its parents' schedule. Invariably people of all ages sharing the same house influence each other's rhythms.

## THE SCIENCE OF SLEEP

Until recently sleep—the "dark" side of our sleep-wake rhythm—was unexplored scientific territory. Some researchers put motion detectors under mattresses to monitor movements during sleep or measured how bright a light or loud a noise had to be to waken a sleeper. Yet it wasn't until the development of sophisticated technology to monitor brain waves (with an electroencephalograph), eye movement (with an electroculograph), and muscle activity (with an electromyograph) that scientists gained real insight into what happens while we sleep.

The biggest breakthrough came in 1954, when researchers at the University of Chicago identified the characteristic pattern of REM or dream sleep. For the first time they had tangible proof that sleep was an altered form of consciousness far more complex than anyone had ever guessed. Their discovery marked the birth of a new biomedical discipline: sleep science.

In the last three decades, the field has exploded. In 1970 only one center in the United States was dedicated exclusively to studying sleep. Today more than 350 institutions offer some expertise in sleep disorders. The number of sleep specialists has soared from fewer than a dozen to several hundred. And the payoff in better nights and days has been enormous.

Sleep science has helped us learn more about the functioning of the brain, the natural cycles of our bodies, the disorders of the mind, and the fundamental changes involved in aging. But its most important contribution has been the development of new insights into and effective treatments for the problems that haunt the nights and shadow the days of millions of men and women.

**ROUND THE CLOCK**

Sleep researchers aren't the only ones paying attention to our night life. For physicians, the study of sleep has transformed the practice of medicine into a twenty-four-hour discipline. "Sleeping patients are still patients," says one doctor, "with diseases that affect them night and day."

Sleep difficulties sometimes serve as warning signals. Centuries ago Hippocrates observed that "sleep and watchfulness, both of them when immoderate, constitute disease." Much more recently, a six-year survey of a million Americans analyzed by University of California researchers revealed that those who slept less than four hours a night or more than ten had roughly twice the death rate of others.

Symptoms hidden during the day may surface only at night, when the body is defenseless and vulnerable. Chest pain sharp enough to rouse a sleeper is a classic sign of heart disease. Severe stomach pain during sleep may indicate duodenal ulcers. Attacks of nocturnal breathlessness could be the result of asthma, allergies, or chronic lung disease.

Even people who are perfectly healthy as they work and play may be in mortal danger as they dream. When cardiologists examined four seemingly healthy men between the ages of twenty-eight and thirty-three who'd complained of nightime chest pain, they found no daytime abnormalities. But a workup at Stanford's sleep disorders center showed that, during REM sleep, their hearts literally stopped beating. All now wear cardiac pacemakers to protect them from dying before they wake.

Sleep studies also have identified headaches that strike only at night. "Cluster headaches" produce localized throbbing pain above the eye, which may become red, swollen, and teary. For some unfortunates, the excruciating ache always begins in REM sleep, continues for ten to fifteen minutes, and recurs two or three times a night, often for periods of several weeks. The typical targets are men in their prime who tend to fit the profile of hardworking, compulsive Type A's.

A newly recognized sleep malady called fibrositis (see page 109) singles out women as its victims. Symptoms include achiness, stiffness, and chronic daytime fatigue. "It's like having the flu all the time," says Harvey Moldofsky, M.D., professor of psychiatry and medicine at the University of Toronto. "For years doctors told women with these symptoms that there was nothing wrong with them. But we've found that these women sleep very, very lightly. And we've been able to induce the other symptoms of fibrositis simply by restricting deep sleep."

Physicians in all disciplines have realized that they've ignored their patients' sleep for too long. Pulmonary specialist Richard Timms, director of the sleep disorders center at Scripps Clinic and Research Institute in La Jolla, California, recalls his surprise when sleep evaluations of patients with lung disease turned up intriguing links between oxygen deprivation in sleep and mental functions, including memory and attention span.

"This may sound like a ridiculous thing for a clinician who sees hundreds of patients a month to say," he observes, "but I had never fully realized the impact a sleep difficulty can have on the quality of life."

## AND TO ALL, A GOOD NIGHT!

Some people would describe a good night's sleep as a minimum of eight hours of rest. Others would emphasize solid, uninterrupted slumber. The best definition is always subjective. "What matters is how you feel in the morning," says NIMH's Stephen Kennedy. "If you feel refreshed and eager and rested, you've had a good night's sleep."

Unfortunately, getting a good night's sleep isn't as simple as it sounds. You might spend hours anxiously waiting to fall asleep, wake time after time in the night, or drag yourself out of bed in the morning feeling almost as weary as when you got into it. But better nights are possible—if you learn more about what goes on when the lights go off.

The rest of this book will tell you everything you need to know about sleep, including information on:

- How to develop good sleep habits (see chapter 2).
- Creating the best possible sleep environment (see chapter 3).
- Mental maneuvers for putting yourself to sleep (see chapter 4).
- Behavioral treatments for insomnia, such as sleep restriction (limiting time in bed to increase sleep efficiency) and stimulus control (learning to associate the bed only with sleep) (see chapter 5).
- New treatments for age-old complaints, such as snoring and sleepwalking (see chapter 6).
- Better understanding of the many causes of daytime tiredness, including physical and psychological factors (see chapter 7).
- Effective new ways to overcome sleep rhythm disorders, jet lag, and shift changes, including step-by-step directions for using light and foods to tinker with biological rhythms (see chapter 8).
- New insights into how dreams, both sweet and scary, can help solve problems in our daytime lives (see chapter 9).
- Simple self-assessments for determining whether you need professional help and where to turn if you do (see chapter 10).

# CHAPTER 2

# The ABZ's of a Good Night's Sleep: How to Get a Good Night's Sleep

*I*magine a perfect night: The bedroom is quiet, dark, safe, soothing. Relaxed and drowsy, you climb into bed. Within seconds of closing your eyes, you drift off. For seven or eight hours you sleep without interruption, dreaming of your favorite people and places. You waken slowly, stretching luxuriously. Energy hums through your body. You feel completely refreshed, ready for whatever the new day may bring.

Perfect nights are possible, but they usually don't just happen. "No small art is it to sleep," Nietzsche wrote. "It is necessary to keep awake all day for that purpose." Like perfect days, perfect nights require planning. And the time to start preparing isn't when you get into bed in the evening, but when you get out of bed in the morning.

What you do—or don't do—from dawn to dusk has an enormous impact on how well you'll rest from midnight to morning. As Drs. Thomas Coates, of the University of

California, San Francisco, and Carl Thoresen, of Stanford University, observe, "Sleeping well depends on living well. Tense and hectic days make for turbulent and troubled nights."

This chapter describes the basic building blocks of a good night's sleep. Some of the recommendations are so simple that you can use them today and feel the difference tonight. But others require more work. According to sleep experts, it can take five weeks for a new sleep regimen to bring about improvements. Be patient. Perfect nights are worth the time and effort.

## QUALITY TIME

By night, quality matters much more than quantity. According to Stephen Kennedy, Ph.D., of the National Institute of Mental Health, "Six hours of good sleep are worth more recuperatively than eight hours of light or disturbed sleep." Less sleep actually produces more benefits. Limiting the time you spend in bed deepens and solidifies sleep; allowing yourself to doze on and off for many hours leads to lighter, more fragmented sleep.

Your goal should be to sleep only as much as you need to feel refreshed the next day. Don't feel that you have to log eight hours. If five hours are enough to recharge your battery, consider yourself lucky. You aren't an insomniac, just a naturally short sleeper.

To figure out how much time you should be spending in bed, keep a sleep diary (see page 154). Note when you go to bed, when you wake up, how you feel at bedtime and on waking, how long it takes to fall asleep, how many times you wake in the night. Also keep track of how you feel during the day, describing your energy level, mood, and activities. After a week or two, look over your records to find the days when you felt most energetic and pro-

# TEN COMMANDMENTS FOR BETTER SLEEP

1. Keep regular hours.
2. Remember that quality of sleep matters more than quantity.
3. Exercise every day—but not in the evening.
4. Don't smoke.
5. Don't have coffee late in the day.
6. Don't drink alcohol after dinner.
7. Don't nap during the day.
8. Unwind in the evening.
9. Don't go to bed starved or stuffed.
10. Develop a bedtime sleep ritual.

ductive and figure out how much you slept the previous nights. Let that amount become the maximum time you spend in bed.

## SLEEPING ON SCHEDULE

The best way to ensure perfect nights is to stick to a regular schedule. If you sleep late one morning and rise before dawn the next, you can come down with a home-bound version of jet lag. To keep your biological clock in sync, get up at the same time every day, regardless of how much or how little you've slept. While your bedtimes should also be fairly consistent, never force yourself to try to sleep when you're not tired.

Keep regular hours on weekends and holidays as well

as workdays. If you stay up late on Friday and Saturday nights and sleep in the following mornings, you can easily give yourself a case of "Sunday-night insomnia": You get to bed early on Sunday night so that you'll be bright-eyed on Monday morning. You try to sleep, but can't. And the harder you try, the more wakeful you feel. As the wee hours of the morning creep by, you finally fall asleep. When the alarm sounds a little while later, you can hardly move.

If you've put in a string of late nights, don't try to make up for lost sleep minute for minute or hour for hour. Sleep seems to be a self-adjusting system, and if you give it a chance, your body will get as much as it needs. Usually a single good night's rest will put the zest back in your step.

When travel or work throws off your routine, try to maintain some semblance of regularity. Eat your meals at the same times you normally do. Try to get some sleep during your usual bedtime hours. And return to your normal schedule as soon as you can. (Chapter 8 provides information on jet lag and shift work.)


## NAPPING

By one wit's definition, a nap is "any rest episode up to twenty minutes in duration involving unconsciousness but not pajamas." Some people seem to be natural nappers. Napoleon, Thomas Edison, President John Kennedy, General Douglas MacArthur, and John D. Rockefeller all indulged in pajamaless sleep. Winston Churchill, a staunch advocate of napping, declared, "Nature had not intended man to work from eight in the morning until midnight without the refreshment of blessed oblivion."

According to one survey, 42 percent of college students, whose schedules offer the luxury of daytime respites, nap five or six times a week. The older we get, the more we nap. Sixty-to-seventy-year-olds take more than eleven naps a week; virtually all seniors over eighty nap often.

But for many people—particularly insomniacs—naps make sleep problems worse. Even though they may feel refreshing, they can undermine sleep efficiency, so that you end up spending more time in bed, yet sleeping less. After a long afternoon siesta, you may find it harder to fall asleep and may wake more often during the night. A better alternative for insomniacs is to take stress breaks during the day and use these ten-minute time-outs for relaxation exercises or meditation.

Even for good sleepers, it may not be daytime sleep per se but the pause that refreshes. Researchers at Texas A&M University found that simply lying down can be as beneficial as sleeping during an afternoon nap. When forty-five "habitual nappers" and forty-five nonnappers were studied, both groups reported the same amount of mood improvement from napping and from resting without falling asleep.

If your schedule doesn't allow you to get enough sleep at night—perhaps because your newborn cries every few hours or you're on night call—napping can help. While naps don't make up completely for lost sleep, they will enable you to perform, not at par, but much nearer to it than without rest. In a recent study at the University of Pennsylvania, two-hour naps compensated for some deterioration in the performance of volunteers who weren't allowed to sleep for periods longer than that during a period of fifty-four hours. In fact, naps early in that time span, even before the subjects were deprived of any sleep, were the most beneficial, almost as if they had a preventive effect.

## WORKING OUT

Exercise has become the wonder drug of the eighties, boosting our bodies' health and our minds' tranquillity. Not surprisingly, what's good for our days is good for our nights. Athletes seem to get more deep sleep when they work out regularly, and many consider a good night's rest a crucial part of their fitness regimen. As studies with sleep-deprived subjects have shown, too little sleep throws off reaction times, interferes with concentration, distorts spatial perception, and increases sensitivity to pain.

Exercise enhances sleep by burning off the tensions that accumulate during the day, allowing both body and mind to unwind. While the fit seem to sleep better and deeper than the flabby, you don't have to push yourself to utter exhaustion. A twenty-to-thirty-minute walk, swim, bicycle trip or run—the minimum for cardiovascular benefits—will also get you into shape for a good night's rest.

Timing is crucial, though. Don't schedule your exercise session for late evening, when you should be concentrating on winding down rather than working up a sweat. And don't expect early-morning exercise to have any impact on the tensions that build up during the day. The ideal exercise time is late afternoon or early evening, when you can use the break to shift gears from daytime pressures to evening pleasures.

## CAFFEINE AND OTHER STIMULANTS

Caffeine is the most widely used stimulant in this country. Americans drink 400 million cups of coffee a day and get extra doses in tea, cola drinks (including diet colas), and chocolate (see chart, page 29). Some people seem innately more sensitive to even small amounts; others build up a tolerance.

But even when heavy sippers insist that coffee doesn't disturb their sleep, all-night sleep recordings indicate that they do sleep differently. In one study of 230 medical students, caffeine prolonged the time they needed to fall asleep and interfered with their normal sleep stages.

If you're a coffee lover, have your last cup at least eight hours before your bedtime. Its stimulating effects will peak two to four hours later, although they'll linger for several hours more. Late-evening caffeine can make it harder to get to sleep, diminish deep sleep, and increase nighttime awakenings.

Caffeine isn't the only dietary sleep robber. MSG (monosodium glutamate), a seasoning often used in Chinese

---

## WHAT'S YOUR DAILY CAFFEINE CONSUMPTION?

Coffee       ___ cups    @ ___ mg   = ___ mg
(fill in dose from table 1)

Tea       ___ cups    @ ___ mg   = ___ mg
(fill in dose from table 1)

Cola drinks       ___ cups    @ ___ mg   = ___ mg
(fill in dose from table 2)

OTC drugs       ___ tablets @ ___ mg   = ___ mg
(fill in dose from table 3)

Other sources                 ___ mg
(chocolate 25 mg per bar, cocoa 13 per cup)

      Daily Total                  ___ mg

| TABLE 1 Caffeine content of coffee, tea, and cocoa (*milligrams per serving—average values*) | |
|---|---|
| Coffee, instant | 66 |
| Coffee, percolated | 110 |
| Coffee, drip | 146 |
| Teabag—5-minute brew | 46 |
| Teabag—1-minute brew | 28 |
| Loose tea—5-minute brew | 40 |
| Cocoa | 13 |

| TABLE 2 Caffeine content of cola beverages (*milligrams per 12-ounce can*) | |
|---|---|
| Coca-Cola | 65 |
| Dr. Pepper | 61 |
| Mountain Dew | 55 |
| Diet Dr Pepper | 54 |
| TAB | 49 |
| Pepsi Cola | 43 |
| Diet RC | 33 |
| Diet-Rite | 32 |

| TABLE 3 Caffeine content of over-the-counter drugs (*milligrams per tablet*) | |
|---|---|
| Anacin | 32 |
| Aqua-ban | 100 |
| Bivarin | 200 |
| Caffedrine | 200 |
| Dristan | 16 |
| Empirin | 32 |
| Excedrin | 64 |
| Midol | 32 |
| No Doz | 100 |
| Pre-mens Forte | 100 |
| Vanquish | 33 |

Adapted from M. L. Bunker and M. McWilliams, "Caffeine Content of Common Beverages," *Journal of the American Dietetic Association*, Vol. 74, pp. 28–32, January 1979

cooking, can have similar effects. Tyrosine, a substance found in chocolate, Chianti, and cheddar cheese, can trigger heart palpitations in the night. Diet pills contain stimulants that can keep you awake. Other drugs or drug interactions can also disrupt your nights. If you're taking any prescription or over-the-counter drugs, ask your doctor whether they may affect your sleep.

## NO SMOKING

Nicotine may be an even stronger stimulant than caffeine. According to several studies, three-pack-a-day smokers take longer to fall asleep, awaken more often, and spend less time in deep and REM sleep. Because nicotine withdrawal can start two to three hours after their last puff, some smokers wake in the night craving a cigarette.

Researchers at Pennsylvania State University compared fifty adults who had smoked an average of 1.25 packs a day for more than three years with fifty nonsmokers of the same sex and age. During four nights in a sleep laboratory, the smokers required an average of fourteen minutes longer to fall asleep and were awake nineteen minutes longer during the night. In another study of eight 2-pack-a-day smokers who quit, their sleep improved dramatically. Within the first three nights of quitting, they cut the time they lay awake in bed by almost half.

## SOBERING THOUGHTS

Alcohol is the oldest, most popular sleep aid. Although many people are in the habit of having a nightcap before going to sleep, liquor late in the evening may cause problems throughout the night. Even moderate drinking can suppress REM and deep sleep and accelerate the fluctuations between sleep stages. Too much wine with dinner can make it harder to fall asleep, and too much at bedtime can make it harder to stay asleep.

If you drink heavily in the late evening, you'll feel the effects on your sleep four or five hours after you get into bed. As the immediate effects of the alcohol wear off, REM sleep—which alcohol suppresses—intrudes onto other sleep stages, depriving your body of deep rest. You end up sleeping in fragments and waking often during the early-morning hours. Once you're up, you may wish you were anything but conscious: With pounding heart, dry mouth, aching muscles, and a throbbing head, every part of your body may be suffering the wrath of grapes.

Another danger is that alcohol may trigger or aggravate sleep apnea, a respiratory problem that affects 20 percent of the population (see chapter 7). In a study at Gainesville, Florida, twenty healthy men between twenty and seventy years old drank four shots of vodka less than an hour before bedtime. They stopped breathing five times more often—and for longer times—than when they didn't have anything to drink. Alcohol may worsen sleep apnea by relaxing the muscles in the throat and suppressing the awakening mechanism, adding to the time it takes for a sleeper to stir and take a breath.

## SNOOZE FOODS

"I do not know what a brain is, and I do not know what sleep is, but I do know that a well-fed brain sleeps well," the British physician Sir William Gull once observed. As scientists have learned more about the effects of various chemicals on the brain, they've identified foods that make us alert and others that make us drowsy. Proteins, such as meat, are energizers, whereas carbohydrates, such as pasta, are sedatives.

Even proteins that contain L-tryptophan, an amino acid that, in high enough doses, can induce sleep (see page 74), aren't the best bedtime bites. The reason, according to Judith Wurtman, Ph.D., research scientist at Massachusetts Institute of Technology's department of nutrition and food science, is that tryptophan has to compete with the other amino acids in proteins to get into the brain. "It's as if many cars were trying to get to a highway on the same ramp," she explains. "Tryptophan is like a Volkswagen that can't get through because the other cars are bigger and faster. But if the other cars disappear, it has a clear field."

Carbohydrates "clear the field" by increasing the body's supply of insulin, which removes other amino acids so that more tryptophan can enter the brain. Milk, the traditional bedtime drink, "has too much protein—about 8.5 grams per cup—in relation to its carbohydrate content, which is 12 grams per cup," says Wurtman. The snacks that made her research subjects sleepiest were bananas or English muffins with jelly.

Other people are less scientific in their presleep dining preferences. Marlene Dietrich reportedly chose sardine-and-onion sandwiches before retiring; Teddy Roosevelt preferred milk with a shot of cognac in it. The Burmese ate pollen cakes. A traditional English favorite was a slowly savored large apple. Gypsies allegedly put the juice of a lemon and an orange and two tablespoons of honey in a glass with hot water and sipped it slowly. Balkan mountaineers drank buttermilk half an hour before bed.

Whatever your choice for a nighttime nibble, keep it light. A big meal late at night forces your digestive system to work overtime. And even though you may feel drowsy initially, you'll probably toss and turn through the night. Avoid peanuts, beans, fruits, or raw vegetables, which can cause gas. And stay away from snacks such as pastries or potato chips, which are high in fat; they take a long time to digest.

But dieters should also be careful not to go to bed hungry. A rumbling stomach, like any other physical discomfort, interferes with your ability to settle down and slumber through the night. In laboratory experiments, the less food that rats were given, the less they slept. After six to eleven days of food deprivation, they seemed to stop sleeping at all, perhaps because hunger drove them to stay awake and hunt.

## SLEEP RITUALS

Before you can slide into sleep, you've got to shift gears, leaving behind the worries and woes of the waking world. Even very young children find it easier to make the transition into sleep if they repeat a few activities, such as saying prayers or reading a story, every night.

Your sleep ritual can be as simple or as elaborate as you choose. It might start with some gentle stretches to release knots of tension in your muscles or with a warm bath. Maybe you like to listen to some quiet music, tune in the *Tonight* show, or curl up with a not-too-thrilling book. Whatever you choose, be sure to do the same things every evening—until they become cues for your body to settle down for the night.

If you've had problems sleeping for a while, the rituals meant to calm you down may be having the opposite effect. As you go through the familiar motions of getting ready for bed, you may also start to worry about how or whether you'll sleep. Even before you close your eyes, your bad night will have begun.

If that's the case, change your sleep rituals. Switch off the nightly news show you usually watch, and lay out your clothes for the next day. Rather than reading in bed, write notes in your diary. These subtle changes carry an important message: you're breaking out of your old cycle of sleeplessness and can and will rest easier.

## SOUND OR SILENCE?

A newborn cries in the night. Within seconds, her mother is awake and rushing to her crib to nurse her, while her

## SLEEP-SHATTERING SOUNDS

*NOTE:* Any sound over 70 decibels begins to activate your nervous system; 120 decibels marks the normal pain threshold.

| | |
|---|---:|
| Traffic on a relatively quiet city street | 70–72 decibels |
| Vacuum cleaner | 81 decibels |
| Sports car or truck | 90 decibels |
| Loud power mower | 107 decibels |
| Jet plane on takeoff | 150 decibels |

father rests undisturbed. A few hours later, his beeper goes off. His wife rolls over in her sleep; he bounds out of bed.

Like this couple, we're all sensitive to specific sounds in the night and are much more likely to react to "relevant" noises. But individuals vary a great deal in their reaction to sounds of different intensities. In fact, some people are as much as seven times more sensitive than others. Women are much more likely than men to waken because of noise in the night. And despite their diminished hearing, the elderly are also more sensitive to noise.

At any age, sounds louder than seventy decibels stimulate signals from the nervous system to the rest of the body. Sudden noises will push your blood pressure upward and lower the supply of blood to your heart. If their intensity increases, your pupils will dilate, the muscles of your abdomen and chest contract, and your heart rate quicken.

Decibels alone don't determine whether you'll waken. A soft but significant sound, like a baby's whimper, is more likely to awaken you than a thunderstorm. In fact, a sudden change in the sound level—a motorcycle backfiring in the quiet or your television buzzing as a station goes off the air—will jar you more than a persistent noise.

When you hear a sound also plays a role in how you react. The deeper your sleep stage, the louder a sound must be to awaken you. Also, you're more likely to be awakened by sounds later in the night, after the longest periods of deep sleep. But even if a noise doesn't wake you, it can disturb your sleep by forcing you to shift from deep sleep into a lighter sleep stage. Studies of people living near airports show that they have less deep sleep and waken more frequently in the night.

If noise is an inescapable part of your sleep environment, try comfortable ear plugs or try masking it with the constant sound of a fan, air conditioner, or a recording of surf or a waterfall. One good alternative is white noise, a continuous sound made up of all the frequencies audible to the human ear. It lulls the mind because it's a medium without a message. All you hear is a hum, much like the one your car makes when you zip along the freeway at fifty-five miles an hour. In one study, students listening to white noise fell asleep within fifteen minutes, whereas others listening to classical music or nothing at all took twice as long to doze off.

## TUCKING YOURSELF IN

If you find yourself lying awake worried about the inevitable bumps you hear in the night, you might make a security check before getting into bed. Double-check the locks on doors and windows, the smoke detector, and the burglar alarm if you have one. An extension phone at your bedside can reassure you that help is just a call away. Be sure to keep emergency numbers handy. If you wear glasses, always keep them in the same spot so that you can reach them without fumbling.

Some people can only sleep in a totally dark room—for good reason. Light is one of the body's most powerful time cues, and the early-morning sun can stimulate your brain to full wakefulness long before you want or need to rise. Try heavy draperies or a light-blocking shade. If you must sleep in the daytime, use comfortable eye shades. On the other hand, if blackness frightens you, a soft nightlight will glow just brightly enough to offer reassurance as you rest.

Most people sleep best in a room that's neither too cold nor too warm. The ideal temperature range for good sleep is the mid-sixties. (It doesn't make any difference whether the air is fresh or not.) If the room is cold, you'll stay in bed longer. If it's warm, you'll sleep less and toss more.

## STAYING UP

What if you've got a big day coming up and you want to make sure you'll get a good night's sleep? Going to bed early to get extra rest can backfire. If you aren't sleepy, you'll simply lie awake. If you start worrying about not sleeping, you may get hardly any rest at all.

A better strategy is to get up earlier the day before. "Prior wakefulness," as scientists call it, enhances the quality and quantity of sleep. The longer you stay awake, the faster you'll fall asleep, the more time you'll spend in deep sleep and the longer your total sleep time will be.

Use the same approach after a bad night. Even though you may be tempted to nap, stay upright and active. Be sure to walk or get some tension-relieving exercise. *Don't* go to bed earlier than usual. Wait until you're really tired and then settle down for a long, refreshing rest. In fact, one study demonstrated that forty hours without sleep greatly improved the sleep of severe insomniacs—but only for a night.

# CHAPTER 3

# Once Upon a Mattress: Creating the Perfect Sleep Environment

Playing and praying. Dreaming and scheming. Sleeping and weeping. Snuggling and snoozing. In the third of your life that you spend in bed, you have time for all these and more. Our beds are our most used pieces of furniture, our most personal possessions, our last bastions of privacy in an intrusive age. Bed is where we head when the world is too much with us, when our temperature rises or our head throbs, when we need time to be alone or to be with the one we love most. As the poet Thomas Hood described it, bed can be "heaven upon earth to the weary head."

Bedrooms have served as settings for dramas and dreams. More murders have been committed there than in all the other rooms of the house combined. And some of the greatest works of music, art, and literature were created by reclining artists. John Milton, Charles Darwin, Elizabeth Barrett Browning, Proust, Colette, and Edith

Wharton wrote in bed. Donizetti once composed a new aria rather than leave his cozy bed to retrieve an earlier draft from the cold floor.

But above all else, beds are important because where you sleep affects how well you sleep. While orbiting astronauts and wilderness adventurers have proven that you could rest anywhere if you had to, nothing compares with the comfort and security of your own bed. "The bed is a bundle of paradoxes," Charles Colton once wrote. "We go to it with reluctance, yet we quit it with regret; we make up our minds every night to leave it early, but we make up our bodies every morning to keep it late."

## THE HISTORY OF THE BED

The first "beds" were probably no more than piles of leaves shoved together by cave people and covered by animal hides. Whole families snuggled together on such primitive mattresses, seeking shelter and protection. Nomadic tribes in Persia invented the earliest form of the water bed: goatskins filled with water to insulate them from the cold earth. For four thousand years the Japanese have been sleeping on futons, thin cotton-filled sleeping mats laid out on the floor at night and rolled up during the day. (A much thicker modern version has become popular in America because it can be stashed in a closet for instant use by overnight guests.)

The Old Testament describes Queen Esther's bed as luxurious, but it simply consisted of a pile of cushions on the ground. Most people of biblical times slept on low tables with wooden headrests. "Mattresses" were stuffed with grass, leaves, twigs, and furs—along with the vermin that nestled among them.

The noble and wealthy eventually devised more ornate places to lay their heads. Egypt's young King Tutankhamen had an exquisite bed made of ebony and gold. The lords of Babylon and Assyria slept on bronze beds encrusted with jewels. The Greeks created elaborate bedsteads of laced hide strips, topping them with animal pelts.

Nero, emperor of Rome, adorned his bed with precious stones purported to have beneficial powers. Other Romans preferred cradle-shaped beds with two chambers—one filled with water, the other covered with a mattress. First they'd lie in the warm water, until, rocked by a servant, they became drowsy. Then they'd move onto the mattress to be rocked gently to sleep.

The fall of Rome set the evolution of bedding back by several centuries. During the Dark Ages even the wealthiest families had to huddle through the nights on piles of animal skins. Medieval man devised more substantial beds, primarily for safety's sake. Many had heavy walls, sliding doors, and hanging night-lights. And while peasants often slept on pallets of straw, aristocrats spent more money on their beds than on any other piece of furniture.

Over the centuries, beds grew in size as well as in spendor. Some were so big that sleepers needed special staircases to climb into them. The famous Great Bed of Ware in England, now on display at the Victoria and Albert Museum in London, was twelve feet square, stood seven and a half feet off the ground, and could accommodate sixty-eight inn guests. In many smaller households, the bed was the most prized possession, handed down through the generations.

Beds shared in the glories of the Renaissance. French and Italian artisans used lightweight inlays and veneers to create delicate details and striking designs. Mattresses also received more attention, as sumptuous velvets, brocades, and silks were used to cover sacks stuffed with pea shucks, straw, or feathers.

During the seventeenth century, Louis XIV, the "Sun

King" of France, transformed his morning rising from bed into a state ceremony. He reportedly owned more than four hundred ornate beds and held audiences and supervised state proceedings from them.

As French aristocrats imitated their king, entertaining from bed became a fad. Beds became so elaborate that some were equipped with built-in heaters and other luxuries for the comfort of visitors. Cardinal Richelieu actually refused to leave his bed when traveling. If his host hadn't made the necessary preparations, the cardinal's men would break down walls, doors, and windows to make room for his mobile mattress.

With the French Revolution, bedding returned to more Spartan standards. Mattresses, stuffed with straw or down, were placed atop a latticework of ropes, which required regular tightening—a practice that led to the expression, "sleep tight."

In the late eighteenth century, Dr. James Graham of London, who had studied the new science of electricity in Philadelphia, hypothesized that the pleasures of the marital union might be intensified if performed under the "glowing, accelerating and most genial influences of the heaven-born, all-animating element or principle, the electrical or concocted fire."

Graham designed a "Celestial Bed" at a cost of eighteen thousand pounds. It was intricately carved, covered by costly silks, and scented with Arabian spices. Mounted on six massive glass pillars and charged with electric currents, it swung rhythmically with the movement of its occupants. Couples eagerly shelled out fifty pounds a night to sleep on this fantastical contraption.

The Industrial Revolution ushered in a new era of bed construction. The invention of the spring provided a new level of support for mattresses, which usually contained cotton, horsehair, feathers, or "shoddy"—wood shavings and other scrap material. Eventually the bedspring evolved into the innerspring construction widely used today.

The development of synthetic rubber in the 1940s led to the creation of the first latex foam mattresses. When a synthetic plastic called polyurethane was developed in the 1950s, this "foam rubber" virtually replaced latex. It's now the most widely used cushioning material in the world.

Most of today's bedding combines innerspring support with the cushioning of foam and natural and synthetic fibers. While contemporary beds might not be as stylistically opulent as those of Louis XIV, they're far more comfortable. And with layers of extra-plush cushioning, luxurious fabrics, and deep support systems, they still qualify as fit for a king.

## BED BASICS

"The bed has become a place of luxury to me," Napoleon Bonaparte once said. "I would not exchange it for all the thrones in the world." Most of us feel the same way, yet we know very little about the furniture we use most.

What makes a bed comfortable and durable is the combination of a quality mattress and matching foundation: a sleep set. To give you the best possible night's rest, this set should provide four fundamental qualities: support, comfort, space, and durability.

• *Support.* Ideally, your spine should maintain the same contours as when you're standing upright with chin, stomach, and pelvis tucked in. If you sleep on a mattress that is too hard or too soft, your muscles must work constantly to straighten your spine. This tug-of-war between mattress and muscle can interfere with your sleep and leave you with a morning backache. According to the American Academy of Orthopedic Surgeons, inadequate support from a mattress, coupled with poor

# WHAT TO LOOK FOR IN A BED

You may think that all beds look alike or that it's almost impossible to tell what you're buying. That's not true. Here are some hints to help you recognize better bedding when you see it:

- *Eye appeal.* Tailoring on quality bedding, like that for quality clothing, is generally superior. Fabrics are usually damask, a high-sheen cloth with a woven pattern, or lustrous knits. The surface may look and feel plush because of a combination of quality fabric and stitch quilting.
- *Thickness.* The mattresses at the very top of the line—and price range—are visibly thicker because they offer lots of extra cushioning. While you may prefer a harder surface, beware of unusually thin mattresses (less than six inches thick).
- *Solid feeling.* Check out the mattress corners. They should have weight and substance. Sit hard on the edges, which should be solid but resilient. If the opposite side flies up when you sit down, keep moving—to another mattress.
- *Soundless and swayless.* When you lie down and roll around, you shouldn't hear or feel any creaking, bumping, crunching, or wobbling.
- *Quality materials.* If you're getting an innerspring mattress, there should be more than three hundred coils in the full-size model. And you shouldn't be able to feel the tops of the springs. If you prefer foam, make sure the foam has a density of at least 1.8 pounds per cubic foot (higher is better).

posture, lack of exercise, and sudden strain, causes millions of backaches.

While a mattress should be firm, it doesn't have to feel as stiff as a board to provide good support. Most people prefer a combination of extra cushioning on top and deep-down support. Yet even firmness is a matter of feel. Terms like *super-firm* and *extra-firm* are manufacturers' descriptions, and one company's *firm* may be harder than another's *super-firm*. Instead of relying on labels, lie down and let your body do the testing.

Once you're on a mattress, pay attention to the support below the heaviest parts of the body—the shoulders and hips—which tend to sink down more. While a too-soft mattress can cause lower back pain, a too-hard surface may create painful pressure at these spots. Ask about the "anatomy" of different mattresses and the materials used to provide support.

• *Comfort*. No one can tell you whether a bed is comfortable; only you can tell which one feels best to you. Manufacturers offer a range of comfort choices, from the harder surfaces to "soft tops." These offer extra layers of cushioning materials, often with an extra layer of super-soft foam quilted to a luxurious fabric. Lie down on a variety of mattresses, including the top-of-the-line models with ultra-plush surfaces, to get a feel for all of your options.

• *Space*. Imagine trying to sleep in a phone booth. That's how a too-small mattress can make you feel. A normal sleeper moves dozens of times in the night, including several full body turns. If you share a bed, both partners need room to roam. Yet two adults sharing a double bed actually have only about as much space as an infant in a crib.

Not surprisingly, more and more Americans are opting for bigger beds. According to one magazine survey, 50 percent of its readers were sleeping on queen- or king-size beds, while almost 65 percent said they would select the larger sizes if they were buying a new bed.

## BED SIZES

These ranges indicate the ideal "comfort zones" for a child, one adult, or two adults.

| | Twin Size 39″ × 75″ | Full Size 54″ × 75″ | Queen Size 60″ × 80″ | King Size 76″ × 80″ | California King Size 72″ × 84″ |
|---|---|---|---|---|---|
| 1 child | _____ | | | | |
| 1 adult | | _____ | | | |
| 2 adults | | | _____ | | |

(The chart above provides a guide to different bed sizes.)

• *Durability.* The quality of the inner construction of the mattress and foundation—the materials and the way they're put together—determines how long the bed will provide maximum support and comfort. Not even the best beds last anywhere near forever. Once your bedding is eight to ten years old, it's no longer providing optimum support and comfort.

The manufacturer's warranty gives you protection against defective materials and poor craftsmanship, but it cannot assure that you'll have the same comfort and support at the end of the warranty period as at the beginning. The best way to assure good performance over many years is to select the highest quality sleep set you can afford.

To ensure maximum durability, purchase a matching foundation with your mattress. It acts as a giant shock absorber, sparing the mattress some wear and tear. In fact, placing a new mattress on an old foundation can reduce its useful life—and diminish the quality of your sleep.

Unfortunately, many people get used to their old mattress's sags and bumps, much as they do to a beat-

# CHECKING YOUR BED

1. Is the cover torn, soiled, or stained?
2. Does the mattress look lumpy?
3. Does the mattress sag where you lie or at the edges?
4. Does the foundation (boxspring) have an uneven, sagging surface?
5. Would you be embarrassed to show your uncovered bed to a neighbor?
6. Does the mattress feel firm and resilient when you lie on it?
7. Is the bed quiet when you turn over?
8. Is the foundation sound and solid (no creaks or wobbles)?
9. Do you and your partner lie comfortably alongside each other without rolling together?
10. Is the mattress still smooth and even to the touch?

Give your bedding one point for each yes to questions one through five and one point for each no to questions six through ten. If your score was between eight and ten, your old bed is definitely ready for retirement. Set aside some time to do a comfort comparison at a local bedding store and select a sleep set that can provide you with a better foundation.

up pair of sneakers, and don't realize that their sleep problems may well be bed problems. If you toss and turn through the night or wake up wincing, give your sleep set the "bed check" above. Since your bed can give out quite gradually, it's a good idea to make this assessment an annual event, particularly after your mattress reaches the eight-to-ten-year-old range.

## TYPES OF BEDS

Because beds now come in so many sizes, shapes, and styles, you have more options than ever before. Here is a guide to what's on the market:

- *Innerspring.* These mattresses and foundations are the most widely purchased type of bedding, accounting for about 70 percent of all mattresses sold today. They use tempered-steel coils for support and are available in a variety of counts and wire thicknesses. Layers of upholstery materials provide insulation and cushioning between your body and the coils. New methods of configuring wire, locking the coils, and stabilizing the springs have led to an almost limitless range of selections.

- *Foam.* Polyurethane foam mattresses, which account for about 10 percent of mattress sales, are available in a variety of densities and foam types, including high-resilience and conventional urethanes. Foam mattresses may have a solid core or consist of several layers laminated together. Support and comfort vary according to the materials.

  While most foam mattresses look alike, the density, resilience, and so-called "comfort factor" can be tailored to meet individual needs. Some foams are so resilient that a steel ball dropped on them will bounce back to 60 percent of the height from which it was dropped.

- *Flotation.* Water beds are hardly a new invention. In 1854, the *Times* of London advertised "Hooper's water mattresses" for "bedsores, fractures, paralysis, spinal afflictions, fever, diseased joints, surgical operations, consumptive and other invalids," adding, "The comfort of these mattresses is greater than can be well conceived."

  After a California student designed the modern water bed in 1967, sleeping on water became a fad for the young, eccentric, and sexually experimental. Since then, water beds have evolved into "flotation sleep systems" that are popular with sleepers of all ages. Today they account for 15 to 20 percent of all beds sold.

Flotation mattresses come in two basic forms: "hard-sides," the most familiar style, consisting of a frame, bag, liner, heater, and platform, and "softsides," which look just like conventional mattresses and foundations. Interior barriers called baffles can provide "waveless" support; modern materials minimize the danger of leaks. A filled water bed weighs thirty-eight pounds per square foot; so, although it is heavy, it weighs less than a refrigerator or twelve adults standing in any room in your home.

- *Adjustable Beds.* These mattresses provide all the basics of conventional sleep sets plus one extra option: They move. New frame engineering and electronic controls have eliminated the institutional look of old-fashioned adjustable beds and transformed them into luxury items that allow sleepers to lift or lower their heads or feet as they read, watch TV, or sleep. Called the Mercedes of mattresses by some manufacturers, these high-priced beds have become especially popular among celebrities.
- *Sleeping on Air.* Introduced in 1980, air flotation beds generally consist of a five-and-a-half-inch-thick air bag, either covered with ticking or set in and topped with foam. Several offer optional electric pumps that allow easy filling and firmness control. Most can be filled with a canister vacuum cleaner or a hair dryer (with the heat turned down or off).

## SHOPPING FOR A BED

Goldilocks may not have realized it, but she was acting like a shrewd consumer when she hopped onto the beds of Papa Bear (too hard), Mama Bear (too soft), and Baby Bear (just right!). The only way to make sure you get a bed that's perfect for you is to do some comparison shopping—and do it lying it down. If, like fifteen million other Americans, you're planning to buy a bed this year, here are tips on what to look for:

- Go shopping only when you're rested and unhurried so that you can concentrate on finding the bed that's right for you.
- Wear loose, comfortable clothes, and shoes you can slip off easily as you try out different beds. For women slacks are better than a skirt.
- Take your bed partner. If you're going to share a bed, both of you should shop for it.
- Shop at stores you know you can trust. Select an established furniture or department store or a specialty bedding store with a reputation for reliability, service, and customer satisfaction.
- Don't just sit on the side of a bed or hop on and off. Lie down and roll around. Get a pillow and lie down with your partner in the positions you normally take to go to sleep. Roll to the center and to the edges. The support should be the same at all points, and there shouldn't be any swaying or creaking.
- Lie on your side for a while to make sure you'll be comfortable in that position. Push down with your hips and shoulders to check how well the mattress will support you. The mattress should push back firmly, but with some resilience.
- Stretch out while lying down. Make sure that the bed is wide enough and long enough so that you're not fighting with your partner for space.
- Stay on the bed for several minutes. If you've been on your feet shopping for a while, any bed will feel good at first. Give yourself time to make a true judgment of comfort.
- Get as much information as you can. Read the brochures and posters. Study any written display material. Ask questions. If the salesman can't answer your questions about the construction of the bed, go to another store.
- Shop for the best value, not the lowest price. While price is important, remember that you're really shopping for the best night's sleep you can buy. Think of your bed as an investment, and go for the best you can afford.

- Buy a foundation that goes with your new mattress. A sleep set will give you maximum support and durability.
- If you and your partner can't agree on the right firmness or size, consider twin mattresses and box springs that share the same frame. A specially designed insert that fits between the two mattresses can eliminate any gulf between you.
- Once you've bought your new bed, get rid of your old one. If it wasn't good enough for you, it isn't good enough for your kids, guests, or neighbors. Some retail stores will pick up and dispose of your old set, or tell you whom to call. A local charitable group may be able to use it in their material recycling shop.
- Don't forget accessories. In addition to a new mattress and matching foundation, you may need a new bed frame, particularly if you're buying a larger set. And don't overlook your need for a protective mattress pad.

## NOW I LAY ME DOWN TO SLEEP

Sleep can bring out a host of idiosyncrasies. Vincent van Gogh would sleep only on a pillow stuffed with hops. Believing that heat interfered with rest, Benjamin Franklin kept at least two beds in his freezing-cold bedroom and moved to the second when the first got too warm. Charles Dickens carried a pocket compass so that he could align his bed due north and south and benefit from the flow of magnetic currents between the poles.

Lawrence of Arabia gave up beds entirely and slept in a sleeping bag of sorts. Sarah Bernhardt allegedly slept in a coffin—a fetish shared by a man from San Francisco, who reportedly spent half an hour in his wife's room each night but could only fall asleep in an open coffin in the next room.

Most people's preferences aren't quite as eccentric, but each of us creates a bedroom that reveals something about ourselves. But you shouldn't worry about what your bedroom says about you; concentrate on creating an environment that will soothe you through the night and into the day. Several accessories may help:

• *Pillows.* Just as your sleep set should support your body in the same posture that it would be if you were upright, your pillow should support your head so that it is in the same relation to your shoulders that it would be if you were standing. A too-thick pillow will strain your neck muscles; a too-thin one will let your head sink.

Traditionally, goose down has provided the best filling for the plumpest—and priciest—pillows. Most of today's feather pillows also include feathers from ducks, chickens, and turkeys and last for ten years or more. Many people prefer pillows made with synthetic fibers. The newest ones provide the feel of down without the high price tag or the potential for allergic reactions. They last about five years.

While conventional pillows are rectangular, you can buy ovals, circles, squares, or triangles. One new model is molded to conform to the shape of your neck. If you like to scrunch up your pillow and burrow into it, stick with traditional shapes. If you have neck or back problems, ask your doctor whether or not a special pillow may help.

• *Linens.* The days of all-white bedding are long gone. Designers have splashed the brightest of colors and boldest of patterns over sheets and pillowcases. You can sleep between purple, plaid, or paisley sheets made out of linen, cotton, silk, satin, or synthetic materials. Even though you close your eyes on these vivid hues, the colors you choose can affect your mood before and after sleep. Some people find tranquil blues and greens especially soothing; others prefer to waken amid sunny yellows and oranges.

While silk or satin sheets may seem like the ultimate in sensuality, you may find them slippery, and they do need special care and laundering. Whatever fabric you prefer, make sure your sheets are smooth and clean.

- *Fleece underblankets.* These woolen underblankets, which lie on your mattress, beneath your bottom sheet, are not like conventional mattress pads. They provide an extra layer of cushioning—thick, soft fleece—and allow air to pass freely around your body, keeping you cooler in summer and warmer in winter.

Ultimately, the best sleep environment is the one that makes you feel best. If you sense that something's amiss or missing, you won't rest well. That's why you should give extra attention to the place where you sleep. Make sure that it's right for you—a room that will cradle you in comfort all night long.

# CHAPTER 4

# 101 Ways to Put Yourself to Sleep

Some of life's longest hours are spent at the edge of night. You lie in bed, longing for sleep. Try as you might, you can't relax or turn off your overactive mind. But you don't have to panic—or reach for a pill to pop. You can put yourself to sleep, naturally and quickly, by using relaxation and focusing techniques. The next time you're stranded in the twilight zone between wakefulness and sleep, relax: *You know how to escape.*

This chapter contains a wide variety of strategies that can help you put yourself to sleep. Some will help your tensed-up body unwind. Others will distract your racing mind. If you're highly visual, those that involve scenes and images may help the most. If you like numbers, playing mathematical mind games may be more effective. Pick and choose different strategies on different nights. Don't work too hard at any, but concentrate fully on each task:

*1.* Tense the muscles of your toes. Hold for several

seconds. Relax. Move up to your feet and lower legs, tensing and relaxing those muscles. Next, gradually work your way up your body: Do your thighs, pelvis, back, chest, shoulders, neck, hands, arms, face, and scalp. Then work your way back down to your toes.

2. Imagine yourself writing perfect numerals six feet high on a make-believe blackboard. Start at one hundred and count backward to zero.

3. Study your surroundings. Count ceiling tiles or floor boards. Carefully examine the construction of your headboard or bedside table.

4. Try to remember a poem you memorized in school, all the verses of the national anthem, or a Christmas carol.

5. Count sheep—or ducks, or peacocks, or zebras. You can distract both halves of your brain by conjuring up a detailed picture of how they look while counting how many are skipping through your mind.

6. Get a tape recording of a monotonous, soothing sound and listen to ocean waves or raindrops as you drift into sleep.

7. Imagine a stroll through your neighborhood, looking at each house, recognizing familiar landmarks, greeting the people you know.

8. Stretch your entire body. Push your arms above your head, point your toes, and stretch till you're as tall as you can be.

9. Turn your air conditioner to the "Fan" setting or buy a white-noise machine and let the sound of static lull you to sleep.

10. Get up. Go into another room and read until you're drowsy. When you return to bed, allow yourself ten minutes to fall asleep. If you're still awake, get up again and return when you're sleepy.

11. Concentrate on inducing a feeling of warmth

or heaviness in different parts of your body. Tell yourself, "My fingers are getting warmer and heavier. I can feel the sensations spreading to the palms of my hands," and so on.

12. Pretend you're Noah, preparing for the boarding of your ark. Think of all the types of animals you're bringing aboard.

13. Play alphabet games, listing girls' names, boys' names, states, countries, trees, flowers, foods, presidents, animals, and so on, in alphabetical order.

14. Make long strings of words by changing one letter at a time: *mind, mild, mold, mole, mile, mill, hill, pill, pile,* and so on.

15. Talk to yourself. Use sleepy words, such as *relaxed, calm,* and *peaceful.* Say, "I am relaxed, I am falling asleep, I feel so peaceful, soon I'll be asleep."

16. Arrange your random thoughts into logical groups. Don't stop to analyze them; just "chunk" them together into categories such as "work" or "children" or "chores."

17. Imagine yourself painting a tall, long wall with a tiny brush. Count your strokes as you dab on the paint.

18. In your imagination, take your favorite walk at your favorite time of day in your favorite season, either alone or with your favorite person.

19. Imagine you're a baby in a cradle being rocked gently to sleep.

20. Watch some reruns in your mind: Go back to a favorite moment, experience, or day and relive it, enjoying every detail.

21. Imagine going to the beach. Feel the sun warming your body. Listen to the waves on the shore and the sea gulls overhead.

22. Say *mmmmmm* to yourself, pausing each time you repeat the sound.

23. Light a candle in your mind's eye. Every stray thought is like a breeze that makes it flicker. Concentrate on keeping the flame bright and straight.

24. Go back in time, year by year, decade by a decade, to a familiar place and watch it change.

25. Pretend you're building and decorating your dream house. Start with the blueprints and floor plan and follow every detail right through to hanging the draperies inside and landscaping the outside.

26. Design a new wardrobe for yourself in your imagination. Try a variety of color schemes and styles.

27. Think back on everything you did during the day, starting with getting out of bed, washing your face, and brushing your teeth, and not skipping any details.

28. Imagine you've just won one million dollars in the lottery. Make plans for saving and spending it.

29. Try to recall what you were doing a year ago. Fill in as many details as you can.

30. Mentally visit your hometown—as it was and as it is now. Go back to your schools, church, favorite hangouts, stores.

31. Think black—a black velvet pillow on a black corduroy sofa on a black wool rug in a black room.

32. Repeat, "I am getting sleepier . . . I am getting sleepier . . . I am getting sleepier."

33. Whenever an image comes into your mind, turn it into gray, like an overexposed negative. Let the gray areas take on amorphous shapes as the colors fade away.

34. Count alternating on-off tones, such as the ticking of a clock.

35. Silently repeat series of numbers: One, one, two. Two, two, two, three three. Three, three, three, three, four, four, four . . .
36. Hold your breath for as long as you can. Relax. Repeat.
37. Make yourself as uncomfortable as you can. Then enjoy getting comfortable again.
38. Keep the instruction manuals and warranties from new appliances or cars next to your bed. Read them slowly and carefully.
39. Sing to yourself—silently, for your bedmate's sake.
40. Write mental letters to the people you'd most like to meet.
41. Tell yourself that if you don't fall asleep, you'll have to get up and do an unpleasant chore. (You may have to make good on this threat for a few nights.)
42. Make love.
43. Yawn repeatedly.
44. Recall a dream, and try to get back into it.
45. Try to stay awake. This technique takes the pressure off so that you're no longer trying desperately to get to sleep.
46. Choose a general topic and find suitable word associations in alphabetical order. Example: *farming—animals, barn, cows, dogs, earth, fields, gardens, horses,* and so on.
47. Swim laps in your imagination. Feel the sting of the cold water. Listen to the splashing of your arms and legs. Concentrate on your form and vary your strokes.
48. Silently count down from three hundred and one in sevens.
49. Think of famous people with double initials:

*AA, BB, CC,* and so on: Alan Alda, Brigitte Bardot, Cyd Charisse, and so forth.

50. Count your breaths.
51. Think of your body as being made of blown glass. As you breathe, a white vapor slowly fills it from head to toe. The deeper you breathe, the more space it fills. Keep breathing until your entire body is white, then switch to another color.
52. Go through the Lord's Prayer, the Gettysburg Address, or a familiar poem, mentally crossing out the *a*'s and *e*'s.
53. Imagine you're playing different instruments in an orchestra, performing your favorite piece of music.
54. Play Around the World in Eighty Days with different letters of the alphabet, such as *B* for *Bali, Burma, Boston, Bangkok, Bristol, Belgium, Brussels, Borneo, Bermuda,* and so on.
55. Imagine rowing a boat across a choppy lake, counting each stroke and coordinating it with your breath.
56. Pretend that it's five minutes before the time you have to get up and try to catch a few more winks.
57. Count your blessings. For an interesting variation, try alphabetizing them.
58. Draw a triangle, a square, and a circle in your mind. Create sculptures by arranging them in different positions.
59. Think of names with initials starting *AA, AB, AC, AD,* and so on: Alan Arkin, Alan Bates, Amy Carter, Andy Devine, and so forth.
60. Make up crossword puzzle or Jeopardy clues.
61. Play anagrams (make up other words from the same letters), choosing a long word, such as *photog-*

*raphy,* which breaks down into *pot, path, pray, hot, hag, hop, toy, trophy, toga,* and so on.

62. Think of three-letter words that you can make using all the vowels, such as *pat, pet, pit, pot, put.*

63. Choose a number and figure out if it's prime.

64. Recite the alphabet to yourself—backward.

65. Mentally try backward-forward writing, such as "Madam, I'm Adam," or "A man, a plan, a canal: Panama."

66. Think of words that contain all five vowels, such as *cauliflower.*

67. Pretend you're walking very slowly into warm water. Gradually submerge your body until you feel yourself floating.

68. Have a cup of herbal tea. Good choices include basil, chamomile, rosemary, sage, peppermint, periwinkle.

69. Take five deep breaths and as you count each one, say to yourself, "I'm getting more relaxed, peaceful, and serene. I'm slowly falling asleep." Concentrate only on this message.

70. Soak in a warm bath for twenty minutes.

71. Make a list of your worries in your imagination, fold it into the shape of a paper airplane, and fly it out the bedroom window.

72. Count backward from 342 by 18's as fast as you can.

73. Spell your name, your spouse's, or a celebrity's backward.

74. Pretend you're at a boring lecture, struggling to stay awake. Feel the tiredness and try to fight it off. Finally let yourself give in.

75. Close your eyes. Place your thumbs on your temples and your fingers on your forehead. Rub gently as you try to empty your mind of all thoughts.

76. If your partner is sleeping beside you, count his or her breaths and inhale and exhale in the same rhythm.

77. Imagine a stormy night in the high Sierras. You're snug and warm in a log cabin, nestled under soft blankets before a roaring fire.

78. Draw a white circle on a black canvas in your mind. Stare at it until it becomes a black circle on a white canvas.

79. Imagine carving a huge marble sculpture of the numeral one, then a more elaborate one of the numeral two, and so on. Make each successive sculpture more intricate than the last.

80. Sniff your way to sleep. Sweet scents for sleep include lavender, orange blossom, pine, cherry, violet, and myrrh. Try putting one in a sachet under your pillow.

81. Play soothing music on a radio or a tape recorder.

82. Plant a seed in a garden in your mind. Nurture it carefully as it develops, watching for shoots, leaves, buds, and flowers.

83. Alliterate. Think of sentences like "Amorous Adrienne ached to assauge abashed Adam's anguish" or "Bashful Bertha belatedly bounded to Bertram's buggy."

84. Reach down and gently massage your feet.

85. Eat a snooze snack, such as milk and crackers or an English muffin with jam (see chapter 2 for more suggestions).

86. Roll your pupils upward and try to keep them there after shutting your eyelids. During World War I a neurologist discovered that soldiers who collapsed into deep sleep didn't wake up even after he lifted

their eyelids with a finger—and their pupils were always rolled upward.

87. Think of as many words as you can that end in "-fy."

88. It's the bottom of the ninth in a tie game in the last game of the World Series, and you're up at bat. Hit a homer, and savor every inch of your run around the bases.

89. Imagine a squadron of jungle beasts on guard around your bed, facing outward, keeping a watchful eye on the doors and windows to your room.

90. Plot a trip, street by street, state by state, highway by highway, across a town, state, or continent.

91. Name every city, then every country, that begins with *q, z,* or *y.*

92. Build words letter by letter or syllable by syllable, such as: *an, pan, plan, plane, planet, planetary, interplanetary.*

93. Place a hot-water bottle on your stomach and rest the insides of your wrists on it.

94. Stare, with eyes shut, at the bridge of your nose.

95. Go for the gold. Pick your sport, and see yourself getting ready to swim, ski, jump, race, or hurdle. Feel your body responding perfectly to your commands. Hear the roar of the crowd as you run your victory lap and receive your medal.

96. If you're a soap opera fan, pick a story line and trace it back as far as you can.

97. Reread a favorite novel in your mind. Try to remember as many minor characters as you can. Fill in actual scenes and dialogue.

98. Imagine that it's a balmy summer day and you're lying on your back under a huge old oak tree. As the breeze fans you, you look up and begin counting the leaves in the tree.

99. Pretend you're in the sky-scraping World Trade Center in New York City. Your job is to go from office to office, starting with the top floor, and shut off the lights. Count each room as you flick each switch.
100. Think of the most comforting person in your life—a mother, lover, friend, teacher. Imagine that you're together in a safe, cozy place, watching a fire slowly burn down.
101. Mentally gather your troubles into a large sack. Tie it to a branch of a tree outside and tell yourself you'll retrieve it in the morning.

# CHAPTER 5

# New Hope for Insomniacs: Treatments That Really Work

*The worst things:*
*To be in bed and sleep not,*
*To want for one who comes not,*
*To try to please and please not.*
*—Egyptian proverb*

Tens of millions of sleep-starved souls would agree that sleep problems should head this list of woes. After many centuries, insomnia hasn't lost its sting—nor surrendered its secrets. This common, complex problem is neither a physical disease, like pneumonia or diabetes, nor a psychological disorder, like depression or anxiety. While its roots can be in body, mind, or both, insomnia is a symptom of something gone awry. Unraveling what and why is the key to overcoming it.

Only recently have physicians taken this challenge seriously. For years, most automatically wrote prescriptions for sleeping pills for weary patients. But as sleep specialists have identified and investigated probable causes and possible cures for insomnia, doctors have been paying more attention to their patients' complaints of poor sleep.

Such complaints number in the millions every year. In a survey of five thousand patients at eleven sleep disorders clinics, about 26 percent had "disorders of initiating and maintaining sleep." According to recent estimates, insomnia keeps more than thirty million Americans up nights. But all insomnias are not the same. A consensus conference sponsored by the National Institutes of Health has identified three general categories:

- *Transient:* The most common type of insomnia, this lasts only for a few nights and strikes almost everyone at some point, usually on the eve of a big event, such as a wedding, job interview, or final exam.
- *Short-term:* This type of insomnia, which may persist for a few weeks, generally occurs at times of job- or family-related stress. Accountants may toss and turn during the feverish weeks before the April 15 tax deadline; a grieving spouse may sleep poorly after losing their beloved partner.
- *Long-term:* Chronic insomnia may last for months, years, even decades. One of the most baffling of clinical problems, it can begin in childhood and persist throughout a lifetime (see page 64).

The most common insomnias are the temporary ones, which account for 60 to 70 percent of all complaints of poor sleep. Yet while transient and short-term insomnia may seem like trivial troubles, they often grow into major ones by instilling a fear of sleeplessness that conditions a sleeper to anticipate—and develop—problems in the night.

In fact, this fear—insomnophobia, as some specialists refer to it—may be even more sinister than insomnia, for

it can transform a few bad nights into an endless quest
for rest. The belief that nothing can or will help turns into
a self-fulfilling prophecy.

Some of the sleepless—fortunately, a minority—seem
to be born insomniacs, with subtle physiological abnormalities that disrupt their rest from infancy into old age.
Others seem more vulnerable to troubled nights. But the
most common causes of insomnia are self-created—and
self-correctable. They include bad sleep habits, a poor
sleep environment, and the use of drugs and alcohol.

At least two-thirds of chronic insomniacs—those with
the most severe sleep problems—do improve after treatment at sleep centers. Once they find a way of improving
their sleep even slightly, insomniacs often make dramatic
progress rather quickly. The reason: a renewed sense of
confidence and control.

## BORN TO BE WEARY?

Some people insist that they've never had a good night's
sleep. They may not be exaggerating. Long after most
babies settle down and sleep through the night, some
infants continue to wake every few hours. And disrupted
sleep patterns can persist throughout their lives.

The reason may involve two different governing systems
in the brain: one controlling arousal and the other controlling rest. At bedtime the arousal system has to subside
and allow the sleep system to take over. Some people may
be born with especially active arousal systems or with
inadequate sleep systems so that they can't make the shift
from wakefulness to sleep smoothly. In various studies,
insomniacs have shown definite signs of greater physiological arousal at night. Their hearts beat faster; their
body temperatures are higher; they wake more often.

Some of these differences may start at, rather than

before, birth. When psychologists Stanley Coren and Alan Searleman, of the University of British Columbia in Vancouver, correlated difficulty falling asleep and frequency of night wakings in 1,272 college freshmen with the circumstances of their birth, they found that various complications of delivery—including breech (foot-first) presentation, prolonged labor, low birth weight, and Rh incompatibility—often led to disrupted sleep patterns in infancy and young adulthood.

"An individual with an early history of sleep difficulties is two times as likely to have sleep difficulties later in life than those who didn't," the researchers concluded. "Tendencies toward insomnia may be part of a lifelong pattern."

In another study of one hundred insomniacs, sleep researcher Ernest Hartmann, M.D., director of the sleep laboratory at Lemuel Shattuck Hospital in Boston, found that thirty-three had trouble sleeping as children and had been told by their parents that they were poor sleepers. Occasionally a trauma, such as a car accident, triggered their initial sleeplessness. But for most, sleep problems started gradually and worsened in times of tension, stress, or depression.

These childhood insomniacs didn't seek help until they reached their twenties or thirties, when they became so fatigued that they found it difficult or impossible to work. Psychological tests showed relatively little emotional imbalance, but often indicated a severe and unusual reaction to even minor amounts of psychoactive drugs. This could be another indication of some subtle abnormality in their brains.

Insomniacs are also notoriously bad at estimating how much they've slept. In one study, only 25 percent of insomniacs (as compared with 81 percent of normal sleepers) were able to guess how long—within ten minutes—they took to fall asleep. When asked about their total sleep

time, half of the insomniacs underestimated it by sixty
minutes.

Insomniacs aren't liars. They honestly cannot tell when
they've slept well. "When we awaken them from sleep in
the laboratory, they'll insist they weren't asleep," observes
Wallace Mendelson, M.D., chief of the Sleep Studies Unit
at the National Institute of Mental Health in Bethesda,
Maryland. "They believe they're awake despite all objective
evidence showing they're not. The inability to recognize
sleep may be the essence of their problem."

Researchers speculate that such insomniacs may have
abnormal sleep patterns too subtle for current monitoring
equipment to pick up or that they may suffer from an
imbalance of crucial brain chemicals. One thing is clear:
Whatever the cause of their complaints, they're just as
miserable as those whose symptoms are verified by all-
night sleep recordings.

## ARE INSOMNIACS DIFFERENT BY DAY?

"Pity us! Oh pity us! We wakeful," Rudyard Kipling once
entreated. But insomniacs rarely get much sympathy.
Theirs is an invisible illness. Except for their bloodshot
eyes or dark shadows, insomniacs look just like anyone
else. But they may be profoundly different—by day as
well as by night.

Two physicians who've done extensive research into the
psychology of insomnia—Anthony Kales, M.D., director
of the Sleep Research and Treatment Center at Pennsylvania State University School of Medicine in Hershey, and
Joyce Kales, M.D., director of Penn State's Sleep Disorders
Clinic—believe that patients with chronic insomnia have
another problem too: "inadequate methods of dealing with
stress."

In a study comparing poor sleepers who'd had insomnia for an average of fourteen years with good sleepers, the insomniacs were much more likely to describe themselves as tense, anxious, overly preoccupied, worried, and depressed. Most had experienced one or more stressful life events—the death of a loved one, a change in work status, or health problems—near the time their insomnia began. They also said that they tended to "take things hard" and often felt they had not lived "the right kind of life." They reported four times more attempts at suicide than the good sleepers.

At bedtime, fewer of the insomniacs felt sleepy. Instead, they were preoccupied with sleep, health, death, work, personal problems. And while they tried harder to get to sleep, they ended up more agitated: turning on the lights, getting up, going to the bathroom, eating, drinking, taking pills. They also woke more in the night because of noise, dreams, physical pain, or thoughts about personal problems or the next day's tasks. And while the good sleepers felt rested, alert, and social in the morning, the insomniacs were tired and irritable.

In a revealing study of insomniacs' days, Evelyn Marchini, of the Pacific Graduate School of Psychology in Palo Alto, and Thomas Coates, Ph.D., of the University of California, San Francisco, monitored ten insomniacs and eleven good sleepers for five days, paging them at random times to find out what they were thinking about and doing. The insomniacs spent significantly more time shopping, watching television, relaxing, and thinking passively about themselves and their immediate environment. The good sleepers were busier, more active, more involved with their work and with others. No one knows if the insomniacs' passivity was the cause or the consequence of their poor sleep.

## INSOMNIA IN A BOTTLE

Sooner or later most poor sleepers reach for a quick fix. They take a long swig of alcohol, buy an over-the-counter sleep aid, or ask their doctors for a prescription for stronger sleeping pills. What they don't realize is the price they'll have to pay. As one researcher put it, they're "borrowing sleep, not buying it." As the levels of alcohol or drugs in their blood drop, they go into withdrawal, which shatters their uneasy rest and causes "rebound insomnia."

Ironically, both alcohol and sleeping pills, which promise deeper sleep, have the opposite effect. After drinking or taking a pill, your sleep becomes shallower and more fragmented. You spend less time in REM or dream sleep, and you may waken early in the morning, too tired to get up but unable to return to rest.

Rebound insomnia can develop after just a few nights of drinking or taking drugs. If you start taking larger drinks or doses, the problem only gets worse. According to one national survey, drug and alcohol use causes the insomnia of 12.4 percent of patients at sleep disorders centers. Increasingly aware of the perils of pills, most physicians advise them only for a few nights during a short-term crisis.

"I prescribe pills for a few nights only when patients have reached the point of no return," says Peter Hauri, Ph.D., codirector of the sleep disorders center at Dartmouth University. "They need sleep so badly that behavioral approaches won't work. Often just the reassurance of knowing that there are sleeping pills in the medicine cabinet is enough to help them relax and get to sleep."

But while you may think that sleeping pills are wonder drugs that can add hours of rest to your night, they don't. In fact, according to several hundred studies, they increase sleep time by only thirty minutes. And their mind- and mood-altering effects linger into the next day. "Pills generally make you feel worse rather than better the next day," says NIMH's Wallace Mendelson. Among the residual daytime effects of sleeping pills that researchers have documented are drowsiness, dizziness, memory loss, and poor coordination (which could be dangerous when driving or doing complex tasks).

"Prescription sleeping pills create a window of impairment," observes Cheryl Spinwebber, Ph.D., of the Naval Health Research Center in San Diego. "There is a period of time when you're very hard to awaken and, once awake, your performance—including memory, reaction times, and other cognitive functions—is definitely impaired."

In one test of the impact of sleeping pills on memory, Martin Scharf, M.D., director of the sleep laboratory at the Jewish Hospital of Cincinnati, gave healthy young adults either benzodiazepines (the most commonly prescribed type of sleep medication) or placebos at bedtime. The next day he asked them to recall items on a tape-recorded word list. All did fine, but at checks eight and twenty-four hours later, those who took the drugs had more difficulty remembering the list. Some didn't recall hearing it.

Often sleeping pills are just one ingredient in a drug "cocktail" of medications for hypertension, heart problems, anxiety, or depression. Some of these drugs, such as thyroid supplements, may actually be the culprits causing sleep problems. Drugs—prescription and nonprescription, therapeutic and "recreational"—can lead to so many sleep difficulties that researchers joke that the best treatment for insomnia would be turning patients upside down and shaking all the pills out of their pockets.

For chronic insomnia, pills are never the ultimate answer. "There is no scientific evidence that any hypnotic

# THE PERILS OF PILLS

Chances are you've taken sleeping pills. After aspirin, they're the most widely used drugs in the United States. Each year Americans buy enough pills to put every man, woman, and child in the nation to sleep for several days and nights. Ironically, the regular pill takers often end up sleeping less and complaining more about sleep problems.

"People who take a sleep medication only occasionally shouldn't feel guilty," says Stephen Kennedy, Ph.D., of the National Institute of Mental Health, who notes that prescription sleeping pills do work when taken appropriately— that is, for a temporary problem. Most stop working within three weeks. And there are very real dangers in overrelying on prescription sleep drugs; these include

- Fatal overdoses, particularly if combined with alcohol or other drugs that act on the central nervous system
- Harmful interactions with other prescription drugs
- Interference with breathing in people with chronic respiratory problems
- "Hangover" effects that impair daytime coordination, memory, driving skills, logical thinking, and mood
- Development of physical or psychological dependence
- Development of tolerance, so that the initial dose stops working and larger and larger doses become necessary
- Disruption of normal sleep stages
- Worsening of the initial sleep problem
- Potentially harmful effects on chronic illnesses of the kidneys, liver, and lungs
- Confusion, hallucinations, and other adverse effects in the elderly
- If taken in pregnancy, possible birth defects
- Difficulty awakening to respond to a fire alarm, crying child, or other crisis

Much less is known about the over-the-counter sleep medications that more than 5 percent of Americans purchase each year. None is considered effective "for prolonged use," and all should be avoided if you're pregnant or have a chronic illness.

# DON'T TAKE SLEEPING PILLS IF . . .

- You have a chronic breathing problem. Sleeping pills can interfere with your ability to breathe.
- You have impaired kidneys or liver. Since many sleeping pills pass through these organs, a dysfunction may mean that the drugs will stay in your body much longer than usual.
- You're taking medications for an illness or chronic disease. You may suffer a serious, even life-threatening drug interaction.
- You're pregnant. Some sleeping pills have been associated with birth defects.
- You're over seventy. Your body may require more time to break down and eliminate drugs. The effects of the sleeping pills may linger, causing confusion and interfering with your daytime functioning.
- You've been drinking. The effects of sleeping pills and alcohol are increased, sometimes with deadly results, when ingested together. A comparatively small amount of a sleeping pill can lead to a fatal overdose in an alcoholic.

*How to Sleep Like a Baby*

drug is efficacious for long-term use beyond two to six weeks," say two top sleep researchers, psychiatrists Robert Williams and Ismet Karacan, of Baylor College of Medicine in Houston. But if you've been relying on sleep medications for months or years, don't quit cold turkey. You'll need professional help to wean yourself slowly from your drug dependence.

## "LEARNED" INSOMNIA: NEGATIVE CONDITIONING AT WORK

Sometimes insomnia starts innocently enough: The pain from a skiing accident wakes you whenever you shift sleep positions. Working late for several weeks to finish a big project, you chain-smoke and down cup after cup of strong coffee. Or you get up every few hours night after night to care for a sick child.

After a string of miserable nights, you get into bed more out of habit than in any hope of getting some rest. You're certain you won't sleep, angry because you can't, and afraid you won't be able to function in the morning. Each night, you try harder to get to sleep, yet end up more wide-awake than ever.

Some people seem particularly vulnerable to getting trapped in this self-perpetuating cycle. According to psychologist Hauri, 15 to 20 percent of the population may be biologically predisposed to "learned" or, as he calls it, persistent psychophysiological insomnia.

"They're naturally light or intermittent sleepers who normally have a bad night once a week or once a month," he explains. "In a time of stress, like a death in the family, they may have several nights of poor sleep, and they become so overconcerned about sleep that they can't relax. A vicious cycle starts in which they worry about not sleeping and they can't sleep because they're worried."

After studying twenty-two such patients, Hauri described the typical learned insomniac as being between forty and fifty, more likely to be a woman than a man, and a sufferer of sleep problems for fifteen years. These poor sleepers spend half an hour more in bed than normal sleepers, but they're asleep only three-fourths of that time.

Learned insomniacs appear psychologically normal on most tests. However, they tend to suppress their emotions and avoid intense, overly exciting sensations. Many also have tension-related symptoms, such as headaches, palpitations, cold hands and feet, and low back pain. Insomnophobia is a key ingredient of learned insomnia. "You can only fall asleep when you don't give a damn about sleeping," says Hauri, "not when you're lying there worrying about getting to sleep."

## TREATMENTS THAT WORK

"If you can't sleep, try lying on the end of the bed," Mark Twain once suggested, "then you might drop off." Much of the advice that poor sleepers have gotten over the years hasn't been much more helpful.

Overcoming insomnia involves some detective work to find out when, why, and how your sleep problem started. If you can trace it to a change in shift, a noisy neighbor, or too many cigarettes, you know where to begin. But because insomnia often becomes self-perpetuating, you may need to do more than mend your sleep-shattering ways.

The nonpharmacological approaches outlined below can and do help. According to researchers at Vanderbilt University Medical Center in Tennessee, behavioral treatments, while not "a panacea for a disorder as complex and as heterogeneous in origin as insomnia . . . are at least

# NATURE'S SLEEPING PILL:
# L-TRYPTOPHAN

L-tryptophan is an essential amino acid, a precursor of the brain chemical serotonin, and a natural sedative. Many high-protein foods, including milk and meat, contain tryptophan. However, the amount of tryptophan contained in these foods is too small to induce sleepiness and, as nutritionists have learned, the other amino acids in the proteins block tryptophan's effects in the brain.

But tryptophan supplements "are an effective sleeping aid," says researcher Cheryl Spinwebber, Ph.D., of San Diego's Naval Health Research Center, who's studied their effects in normal and poor sleepers. "In good sleepers experiencing situational insomnia, a dose as small as a gram will help. Chronic insomniacs may need two to three grams and may have to take tryptophan for several nights before getting any benefits."

Unlike other sleeping pills, trytophan doesn't alter the normal biochemistry or stages of sleep, nor does it have any residual effects on daytime functioning. "For most people, I believe it's the sleep aid of choice," says Spinwebber.

Several studies have confirmed that tryptophan increases total sleep time and deep sleep, shortens the amount of time it takes to fall asleep, and decreases the amount of time awake in the night. In one experiment in Switzerland, forty chronic insomniacs took two grams of tryptophan on a three-day-on, four-day-off schedule for about four months. By the end of the study, half said they were sleeping normally, while another 30 percent said that their sleep patterns were "much improved." Two years later, a follow-up study showed that most were no longer taking tryptophan but were sleeping well nonetheless.

> Scientists have some words of caution about regular, heavy use of L-tryptophan, though. Moderate to heavy doses of the amino acid have caused changes in the liver in experiments on animals. No one knows (yet) if these effects also occur in humans, or if they're a serious health threat.

as effective on a long-term basis as hypnotics (sleeping pills) and without question safer."

And don't ever think you're too old to sleep better or to stop resorting to drugs. A recent study of fifty-three insomniacs in their fifties and sixties showed that behavioral interventions definitely improved their sleep. After four weeks, the volunteers felt they were sleeping better and feeling more refreshed in the morning. Perhaps just as importantly, they also felt that they had more control over their sleep.

## SLEEP RESTRICTION

"No wonder you've got insomnia," the writer Peter de Vries once quipped. "All you ever do is sleep." There's wisdom as well as wit in these words. The best way to help insomniacs sleep more may be by forcing them to sleep less.

That's what Arthur Spielman, Ph.D., then at Montefiore Medical Center in the Bronx, New York, and Paul Saskin, Ph.D., of Toronto Western Hospital, concluded several years ago after observing that insomniacs often spend eight or nine hours in bed, even though they sleep for only five or six of those hours. Because they're tired in the day, they're also likely to nap. The two researchers speculated that chronic insomniacs might fall asleep faster and waken less if they weren't allowed to spend so much time in bed.

In an eight-week study at Montefiore, thirty-five poor sleepers—averaging fifteen years of insomnia each—logged their sleep habits for two weeks, recording their time in bed, time of arising, and estimated time asleep. The average amount of time they spent *sleeping* became the maximum time they were allowed in bed. For most, that meant going to bed an average of 140 minutes later and not napping at all.

Based on daily phone reports, the sleep researchers determined how efficiently each insomniac was sleeping by dividing the hours each slept by the time spent in bed. Once they stayed asleep for 90 percent or more of their time in bed for five nights, the volunteers could go to bed fifteen minutes earlier. Those who still weren't sleeping efficiently had to restrict their sleep time even more. After two months, 86 percent of the participants were sleeping longer and more restfully. After six months, most still reported improved sleep, particularly if they limited their time in bed.

## RELAXATION TECHNIQUES

"Relax," friends may say when you complain about sleeplessness. But relaxing is no simple matter, particularly if you are trying to relax yourself to sleep. With practice, you can learn ways to release the tension that tightens your muscles and keeps you awake. Here are the best methods:

### PROGRESSIVE MUSCLE RELAXATION (PMR)
Developed by Edmund Jacobson, M.D., progressive muscle relaxation involves alternating the tensing and relaxing of various muscle groups in the body. You focus on the

muscles of your arm, for example, tensing them tightly for a few seconds and then releasing them. As you focus on the different parts of your body, you learn to recognize how your muscles feel when deeply relaxed. Practice is essential, and you'll become more relaxed more quickly as you become accustomed to the exercise. (See the accompanying box for specific instructions.)

## AUTOGENIC TRAINING
Autogenic training involves concentrating on repetitive phrases (such as "My feet are becoming heavy, my legs are becoming heavy . . .") that emphasize a feeling of heaviness and relaxation in different parts of the body. For example, you might imagine your feet becoming heavy and warm, then let that feeling move up to your legs, then your thighs, then your hips, and so on, until your entire body feels relaxed.

## TRANSCENDENTAL MEDITATION
Revolving around the mental use of a sound, called a *mantra*, Transcendental Meditation can help to bring about a state of alert restfulness. You don't use this technique before bedtime, but during twenty-minute periods in the morning, afternoon, and evening to relieve daytime stress. In one study people who meditated twice a day for six months fell asleep more quickly at night than before they began practicing meditation.

## YOGA
Yoga is an ancient discipline designed to promote physical fitness and mental well-being. It can also help your body and mind to unwind and can ease your way into sleep. Here are two simple exercises you can do in bed:

# PROGRESSIVE RELAXATION

1. Make sure you're comfortable.
2. When tensing your muscles, do so vigorously—but not so vigorously that you develop a cramp. Hold the muscle in its tensed position for five to seven seconds, counting 1,001, 1,002, and so so. Then relax for fifteen to twenty seconds.
3. Concentrate on what is happening. Feel the buildup of tension; notice the tightening of the muscles; feel the strain and then the release; relax and enjoy the sudden feeling of limpness.
4. You will be tensing and relaxing each muscle group twice. If any specific part of your body still feels tense after completing the exercises, go back and tense and relax those muscles again.
5. Try to keep all other muscles relaxed as you work on a specific group.
6. To begin, take three deep breaths, holding each one for five seconds.
7. Clench your right fist if you're right-handed, your left fist if you're left-handed. Hold and count for five to seven seconds. Relax. Repeat.
8. Flex your dominant bicep. Tense. Relax. Tense. Relax.
9. Clench your other fist. Relax. Repeat. Tense your other bicep. Relax. Repeat. Take a couple of deep breaths and notice how relaxed and warm your arms feel. Enjoy the sensation.
10. Tense up the muscles of your forehead by raising your eyebrows as high as you can. Hold for five seconds. Relax. Repeat. Let a wave of relaxation wash over your face.
11. Close your eyes very tightly. Release and notice the relaxation. Repeat.
12. Clench your jaws very tightly and make an exaggerated smile. Release. Repeat.

13. Take a couple of deep breaths and notice how relaxed the muscles of your arms and head feel.
14. Take a deep breath and hold it a few seconds. Release slowly. Repeat.
15. Try to touch your chin to your chest but use counterpressure to keep it from touching. Release. Repeat.
16. Try to touch your back with your head, but at the same time push the opposite way with the opposing muscles. Notice the tension building up. Release quickly. Repeat. Let your neck muscles become completely relaxed.
17. Push your shoulder blades back and try to make them touch. Notice the tension across your shoulders and chest. Relax. Repeat.
18. Try to touch your shoulders by pushing forward as far as you can. Hold. Relax. Repeat.
19. Shrug your shoulders, as if trying to touch them to your ears. Hold. Release. Repeat.
20. Take a very deep breath. Hold for several seconds and release slowly. Do this again, noticing a wave of relaxation overtaking your body.
21. Tighten your stomach muscles and hold for several seconds. Relax. Repeat, noticing the relaxed feeling in your abdomen.
22. Tighten up your buttocks. Hold. Release. Repeat.
23. Tense your thighs. Release quickly. Repeat.
24. Point your toes away from your body. Notice the tension. Return to a normal position. Repeat.
25. Point your toes toward your head. Return to a normal position. Repeat.
26. Point your feet outward. Release quickly. Repeat.
27. Just let your body relax for a few minutes. Notice and enjoy the good feeling.

Practice this routine twice a day. When you become proficient, schedule a practice session for bedtime. Don't worry if you fall asleep before finishing. That's the whole point.

*Tension Reliever*
1. Lie flat on your back. Inhale to a count of five. Raise your arms over your head until your hands touch the bed. Make two fists.
2. Raise your buttocks. Tense and stretch every muscle in your body, including those of your face.
3. Hold for a count of five.
4. Release your breath and relax your body, keeping your arms over your head. Relax your fingers. With eyes closed, let the tension drain out of your body.
5. Repeat, slowly increasing the amount of time you spend in this position by several seconds each day.

*Sponge*
1. Lie on your back, feet slightly apart, hands at your sides, palms upward. Close your eyes. Breathe normally.
2. Check your body for hidden tension in your legs, hands, face, or shoulders.
3. Concentrate on releasing all negative feelings, such as tiredness, restlessness, or tension. Mentally replace these with feelings of lightness and serenity.
4. Relax each part of your body, starting at your toes and working up to your forehead. Do not rush.

## COGNITIVE REFOCUSING
Often insomniacs' bodies are weary, but their minds won't let them rest. Worries, fears, plans, regrets, and ideas crowd into consciousness. Try as they might, they can't turn off their racing brains. Yet that's exactly what cognitive refocusing does. "Many people complain of being overly alert or aroused at bedtime," says psychologist Patricia Lacks, Ph.D., a professor at Washington University. "Cognitive refocusing teaches them to use imagery to focus their minds and allow them to relax."

Among the mental maneuvers you can use to banish

unwelcome thoughts are focusing on minute details in your surroundings, doing math problems, or conjuring up soothing scenes. (Chapter 4 provides dozens of specific strategies.)

*MONOTONOUS STIMULATION*
Another technique for quieting an overactive mind is to listen to a simple, repetitive sound. In sleep laboratories, alternating on-off tones helped people fall asleep faster than total silence or a single unbroken sound. Many people prefer "white noise," a combination of frequencies that produces a constant hum. An air conditioner set at "Fan" provides this effect. Others play tapes or use special machines that sound like ocean waves or raindrops.

*STIMULUS CONTROL*
This technique, developed by psychologist Richard Bootzin, Ph.D., of Northwestern University, is a classic behavioral approach to sleep that's demanding but effective. Its basic premise is to condition yourself to associate your bed with rest. You're not allowed in bed for any purpose other than sex or sleep.
   Here are the fundamental guidelines:

• Go to bed only when sleepy.
• Don't read, eat, watch television, knit, or chat with your partner in bed.
• If you don't fall asleep within ten minutes, get up and leave the bedroom. Don't go back to bed until you feel sleepy. If you don't fall asleep within ten minutes, get up again. Do this as often as necessary until you fall asleep within ten minutes of getting into bed.
• Regardless of how often you commute to and from your bedroom and how little you sleep, get up at a set time.
• Don't nap during the day.

- Keep a careful record of when you went to bed, how often you got up, how much time you spent out of bed.

On the first few nights, you can expect to get out of bed five to ten times and to rest very little. If you're tempted to give up, turn to friends, family, a sleep specialist, or your doctor for support. If you keep conscientious records, you should see signs of improvement within a few nights. Within three weeks, you should be sleeping much better. In six weeks, you should be able to settle down immediately and sleep through the night.

## PARADOXICAL INTENTION

Trying to stay awake can help you fall asleep. It may sound contradictory, but it works. In one study at Temple University, five chronic insomniacs tried relaxation therapies to help them fall asleep, with limited success. Then the researchers told them that they needed more information about their presleep thoughts. Specifically instructed to try to remain awake as long as possible, in order to describe these thoughts better, they fell asleep faster than ever, cutting the time they spent awake before falling asleep by more than 50 percent. One woman who had taken ninety minutes to fall asleep initially and who fell asleep in seventy minutes after trying relaxation techniques nodded off in just five and a half minutes.

Why did trying not to sleep work so well? The researchers speculate that some people see each night as a test and become highly anxious at bedtime. When they don't fall asleep quickly, they start worrying about their deteriorating ability to sleep. Once the pressure's off, they can stop worrying—and start sleeping.

## HYPNOSIS

Although named for Hypnos, the Greek god of sleep, hypnosis is not a state of sleep or unconsciousness. However, hypnosis can help you get to sleep. A psychologist or psychiatrist trained in hypnosis can teach you how to induce a trance, a state of heightened awareness in which you focus your attention on a particular scene or message. The deep relaxation that accompanies the trance can make you drowsy. In addition, the therapist gives specific suggestions that help you overcome your fear of insomnia and make you feel confident that you will sleep. Some troubled sleepers play a tape recording of the hypnosis session at bedtime.

Many people use a form of hypnosis to fall asleep without realizing it. As they lie in bed, they breathe deeply, relax their muscles, and repeat a message such as, "I am falling asleep. I am falling asleep. I am falling asleep." These positive suggestions keep anxiety at bay and help lull you into sleep.


*BIOFEEDBACK*
Biofeedback lets you control various physiological functions by learning to recognize how your mind influences your body. Sophisticated equipment measures muscular tension or brain waves and translates them into visual or audio signals. By concentration, trial and error, and practice, you can bring about physiological changes that affect the feedback signal.

EMG biofeedback equipment measures the electrical currents generated in the muscles, amplifying and converting them to an audible tone. SMR (sensorimotor) biofeedback helps an individual maintain a particular electrical brain rhythm and is more difficult to master.

Peter Hauri, of Dartmouth, has found that both EMG and SMR biofeedback can help certain patients. EMG biofeedback reduces complaints about sleep in people who are tense or hyperaroused. SMR biofeedback, most often used in experiments with individuals who wake in the night, helped insomniacs who were not tense.

## PUTTING INSOMNIA TO BED

No one can guarantee insomniacs that they'll never have another sleepless night. But they can have many more good nights. The secret isn't a miracle cure, but a combination of good sleep habits and various behavioral approaches.

"I've found that the secret of helping the patients who come to our center is tailoring the therapy to each individual," says psychologist Hauri. "I want to know everything that happens during the night in minute detail. If someone is looking at the clock every few minutes, I may suggest that he get rid of it. If he's tense, I may suggest distracting techniques. If he's spending too much time trying to sleep, I may tell him to get out of bed. No one treatment will work for all insomniacs, but a combination of different ones can help."

If you're wide-eyed when you wish you weren't, develop a systematic strategy for improving your sleep. Follow the guidelines for good sleep habits in chapter 2 and for creating a good sleep environment in chapter 3. If your mind keeps racing like a revved-up engine, experiment with the mental exercises described in chapter 4. If your body feels tense, try the muscle-relaxing techniques in this chapter. You, too, may find that no one approach works every night, but the right combination may pay off, not just for one night, but for the rest of your nights.

# CHAPTER 6

# Making It Through the Night: Problems Staying Asleep

All across the country, the night is anything but still or silent. A shift worker in Detroit comes home at 2:00 A.M. to find that his wife and three children have sleepwalked into the kitchen and are eating breakfast. An intern in Los Angeles who collapses onto her bed after thirty-six hours on call mumbles medical orders as she sleeps. A slumbering salesman in New Jersey grinds his teeth so vigorously that he's wearing away the enamel. A visiting grandmother in Florida wakes up her son's family with her ear-splitting snores.

These less-than-serene sleepers are hardly unusual. Some four million Americans regularly stroll in their sleep. As many as one in every five talks in his sleep. Millions more grind their teeth, flutter their legs, or shatter the silence with their snores. While some nighttime disruptions, such as babbling, are mere nuisances, others, like sleepwalking, can endanger life and limb.

Some of these sleep disorders are related to each other. Sleepwalking, sleep talking, bed-wetting, and night terrors—all problems of partial arousal, or parasomnias—strike people who spend more than the usual amount of time in the deepest stages of sleep. They're also hereditary, so if you have one, you're at risk of developing others! This chapter will tell you how to recognize the problems that interrupt your sleep and what you can do to overcome them.

## SNORING

"Laugh and the world laughs with you, snore, and you sleep alone," the writer Anthony Burgess once observed. For millions of snorers and their sleep-starved partners, snoring is no laughing matter. One of every eight people snores, with men outnumbering women by four to one.

When small children snore, enlarged tonsils and adenoids are usually the culprits. Teenagers and young adults tend to be silent sleepers, with the incidence of snoring in both sexes increasing steadily after age thirty. According to David Fairbanks, M.D., of George Washington University, 20 percent of men and 5 percent of women between the ages of thirty and thirty-five snore. By age sixty, 60 percent of men and 40 percent of women are habitual snorers.

Snoring is the result of the blockage of an air passage during sleep. The vibration of the soft palate as the lungs struggle for air creates the rattles and roars. The most common causes are excessive fatty tissue in the throat, large tonsils, or a deviated septum or other deformity of the nose. Snoring is three times more common in obese individuals than in thin ones. Eating, drinking, or heavy smoking before bed also tend to increase snoring.

You're most likely to snore while lying on your back

## FAMOUS SNORERS

George Washington
Abraham Lincoln
Theodore Roosevelt
Franklin Delano Roosevelt
Beau Brummel
Plutarch
Winston Churchill
Benito Mussolini

because your tongue may fall over your throat, interfering with the air flow to your lungs. The resulting sound can be quite an earful. Researchers have recorded snores as loud as eighty decibels. That's as loud as the sound of a Greyhound diesel engine heard from the rear seat of the bus.

Most snoring is only an occasional nuisance, but nightly snoring can be extremely serious. The obstructed flow of air stresses the heart and lungs of snorers, leading to premature high blood pressure. Loud snoring may also be a sign of a severe, potentially deadly problem: sleep apnea, a condition in which breathing stops periodically for seconds or even minutes (see page 113).

The noisy snores of a person with sleep apnea echo through the house, and they're punctuated with silences. The pauses are the periods during which breathing stops; gasps and snorts accompany the sleeper's struggle for air. In severe cases, medical or surgical treatment is essential to eliminate the risk of sudden death during sleep. If you or your partner bellows regularly through the night, check

# HOW TO STIFLE A SNORER

- Humidify your bedroom. Dry, swollen mucous membranes may block air passages.
- Don't drink or smoke. Both alcohol and nicotine can inflame and swell mucous membranes, but it may take two to three months of abstinence before you notice any benefit. At the very least, don't drink or smoke for three hours before going to bed.
- Lose weight. Fat, flabby muscles in the mouth and throat are prime culprits in setting off snores.
- Sleep on your side rather than on your back. To keep from rolling over, fasten a pillow around your middle with a belt or put a marble or golf ball in a small pocket in the back of your pajamas. During the American Revolution, soldiers sewed metal "snore balls" into the backs of their sleep clothing. An easy alternative is to put a tennis ball in a sock and pin it to the back of your pajamas.
- Check with your doctor to see if you're allergic to house dust, the feathers in your pillow, pollen, or other common substances. Allergens can swell mucous membranes, so hay fever sufferers who sneeze throughout the day may snore throughout the night.
- Be wary of antisnoring gadgets, such as chin straps, face masks, head braces. Although they can keep your mouth shut and prevent your jaw from falling back, they may be too uncomfortable to sleep in.
- Check with your family doctor or an ear, nose, and throat specialist to see if you have enlarged tonsils or a crooked nasal septum.
- Exercise. By shaping up, you'll lose weight and tone your muscles, including those in your throat.
- Don't take sleeping pills, antihistamines, or tranquilizers—they can interfere with normal breathing.

- Elevate the head of the bed. Try putting a brick under the bedpost.
- Try visualizing yourself sleeping silently—mouth closed, lying on your side—and repeat this mental rehearsal several times during the day.

with your physician or a sleep disorders center. There may be more to the problem than meets the ear.

For most snorers, the simplest solution is rolling onto their side or stomach so that gravity pulls the tongue forward and down, making room for air to pass through quietly. If you snore and can't resist lying on your back, raise the head of the bed by putting pillows under the mattress or a brick under the bedposts (or try the other practical tips in the chart above). Stay away from "antisnoring" devices that try to muzzle your mouth.

Some desperate snorers have tried more elaborate treatments. In one experiment, researchers hooked up a sound-sensitive monitor to six snorers so that they woke up when they began to sound off. After two weeks, all six were snoring less. David Fairbanks, M.D., an ear, nose, and throat specialist, studied forty-two snorers who underwent major surgery to clear blocked nasal breathing passages and change the shape of the tissues in their throat. The operation—technically known as uvulo-palato-pharyngo-plasty (UPPG)—reduced snoring in 77 percent of the patients.

Snorers often slumber peacefully through the din they create; their weary bedmates are the ones with sleep problems. If your partner rumbles all night long, try to fall asleep before he or she does. Wear earplugs to bed, or turn on the radio or a tape recording of monotonous sounds to camouflage the noise. Some researchers tried conditioning snorers' wives to the sound. Every evening they played a tape of a husband's snoring as the wife fell asleep, starting off low and gradually turning up the volume. Over a two-week period, the wives were able to sleep peacefully, oblivious to their spouse's snores.

## SLEEPWALKING

About 2.5 percent of adults sleepwalk regularly. Children are far less likely to stay under the covers. Between the ages of five and twelve, 10 to 15 percent of children— with boys outnumbering girls—walk in their sleep at least once; 6 percent leave their beds once a week or more.

Doctors don't consider somnambulism (sleepwalking) a disease or a clear-cut symptom of disease. However, it can be deeply troubling, not only to those who walk or talk in the night but to partners and parents as well.

For centuries people believed that evil spirits bewitched unlucky sleepers and forced them to roam through the night. Many still think that sleepwalkers are acting out their dreams. However, our muscles are paralyzed while we dream, and we cannot move. Sleepwalking always occurs during the deepest stage of dreamless sleep. In unknown ways, a malfunction of the brain's sleep control system propels an individual from profound rest into a state of partial physiological arousal.

Heredity makes some individuals particularly vulnerable. According to Anthony Kales, M.D., professor of psychiatry and director of the Sleep Research and Treatment Center at Pennsylvania State University School of Medicine in Hershey, the closest relatives of a sleepwalker are ten times more likely to become night wanderers than the general population. William Dement, M.D., director of the Sleep Disorders Center at Stanford University, tells of one patient who awoke in his grandfather's dining room

# HOW TO KEEP A SLEEPWALKER SAFE

If you or someone you love prowls through the night, take the following precautions to prevent accidents and injuries:

- Remember that regular hours and afternoon naps (which reduce deep sleep during the night) can help both adults and children sleep peacefully through the night.
- If possible, have the sleepwalker sleep on the ground floor so that he won't fall down stairs or out a window. If that can't be done, install protective gates across the bedroom doorway. Block all stairways so that he can't go up or down them.
- Lock windows and doors to the outside and keep the keys with you.
- Hide knives, other dangerous objects, and car keys. Remove all firearms from the house.
- Answer a small child's questions about sleepwalking frankly, but don't call excessive attention to it. With older children or adults, discuss safety measures and make it clear that you are trying to protect, not punish or embarrass, them.
- If you come upon a sleepwalker, try not to startle him. If possible, lead him gently back to bed without waking him.
- If you must arouse a sleepwalker because he is in danger, don't yell, slap, or shake him or splash cold water on his face. Repeat his name calmly until he shows some signs of response, then reassure him that he's okay and guide him back to bed.

> • Folk remedies, such as a pan of water at the sleepwalker's
> door or a rope tied around his waist, usually don't work.
> Sleepwalkers seem to have selective powers of perception
> and often learn to step over the pan or untie the knot
> in the rope.

in the middle of the night at a reunion to find himself
surrounded by sleepwalking relatives.

Children are the most frequent sleepwalkers. Their still-
developing central nervous systems may not be capable of
making a smooth transition from one sleep stage to
another. A seizure disorder, high fever, or extreme fatigue
also can pull youngsters to their feet. Occasionally, the
mind plays a greater role than the body.

"School-age children may sleepwalk because of psychological factors," says Richard Ferber, M.D., director of the
Center for Pediatric Sleep Disorders at Children's Hospital
in Boston. "Generally these are delightful, well-behaved
kids with deep negative feelings bottled up inside. Often
they're living in an environment over which they don't
have any control, maybe because of a divorce or an illness."
Such young night strollers tend to sleepwalk more often
than other children and appear more agitated when they
do.

If you discover that your child sleepwalks, the best
approach is a low-key one. "Too often I see parents who
say, 'My child is weird because he sleepwalks,'" Ferber
says. "That's a very bad message to give to a youngster,
and it's not true. Lots of children walk in their sleep, and
most outgrow it by their teens with no physical or emotional
aftereffects."

While Ferber advises ignoring an occasional episode, he
adds, "If an older child is sleepwalking more and more

frequently, consult your pediatrician, who can refer you to a sleep specialist to evaluate everything that's going on." An all-night polysomnogram (a recording of the brain's electrical activity during sleep) can pinpoint or rule out a seizure disorder. In some cases, psychotherapy may be recommended to help a troubled child confront and express painful emotions.

"Sleepwalking in adults is a totally different animal than it is in children," says Dr. Wallace Mendelson of the National Institute of Mental Health. "Unless a seizure disorder or the use of hypnotic drugs is the cause, most cases are related to some psychological disturbance, which can range from mild to severe. I'd suggest seeing a psychotherapist, who can evaluate the situation and recommend treatment that will address the source of the stress or the underlying psychological problem."

In a study of twenty-nine adult sleepwalkers, Kales and his colleagues at Penn State found that most started their midnight rambles after a major life crisis and roamed more often during times of stress. Through in-depth interviews, they also discovered that 72 percent had psychiatric problems, usually involving feelings of extreme anger in dealing with frustration, failure, or loss of self-esteem.

Many sleepwalkers do nothing more than sit up or stand by their beds for a few minutes. Even those who go longer distances usually return to sleep within thirty minutes and wake in the morning with no memory of where they've been or what they've done. While movies show sleepwalkers tiptoeing nimbly along narrow window ledges, threading their way across busy highways, or climbing unscathed up and down ladders, real-life night explorers can and do hurt themselves. According to sleep researchers, 72 percent of adults and 33 percent of children who sleepwalk have suffered injuries ranging from bruises as a result of collisions with furniture to broken limbs due to tumbles down stairs or through open windows.

While they're rarely violent, sleepwalkers can harm others and the things around them. A sleepwalking man hit his wife over the head with a lamp; another caused an explosion when he tried to heat a bottle of vodka on the stove. One somnambulist put the good china in the clothes washer and woke up as the machine crunched the expensive dishes to smithereens. Several years ago a woman murdered her daughter during a sleepwalking episode triggered by a sleep-inducing drug.

Adults who sleepwalk often, over a period of six months to a year, should see their family doctor, who can refer them to a sleep specialist for a polysomnogram or, if indicated, to a psychiatrist for help in dealing with underlying psychological difficulties. If stress is the problem, simple relaxation therapies, such as biofeedback and progressive muscle relaxation, can reduce both daytime tension and nighttime restlessness. Hypnosis has helped some roving adults by teaching them to wake up whenever their feet touch the floor.

In extreme cases of frequent sleepwalking and a serious risk of injury, doctors may prescribe drugs that reduce deep sleep, such as Valium (a tranquilizer) or Dalmane (a sleeping pill), usually in the lowest possible doses for the briefest possible time. "But they're not supereffective," says Mendelson, "so it's always much better to address the real source of the problem."

## SLEEP TALKING

Chances are you've talked in your sleep; we probably all have. But what we say isn't worth waiting up to hear. Sleep researchers consistently report that they've never heard sleepers say anything in their sleep that they would be ashamed to say while awake. Rather than revealing dark secrets, sleep talkers make little, if any, sense.

Most sleep talking occurs during the lightest stages of sleep and consists of a few brief words. Someone who's just fallen asleep may respond simply to queries, but true conversations are rare. More often than not, sleep talkers seem to be muttering words such as *okay* or *gee* to themselves.

Only 10 percent of sleep speech occurs during dreams, and the talkers' words can provide some clues as to what they're dreaming about. One man in a sleep laboratory said, "Argentina's a long way away." Awakened, he recalled dreaming of a woman he'd dated the previous summer who was from Argentina. Another person asked, "What do you think whales eat?" He reported a dream about people on boats who were being chased by whales.

Sleep specialists don't consider sleep talking a sign of psychological or physiological disturbance. One describes it as no more than a "benign quirk." If you babble in the night, you needn't wory about shameful revelations. If you're the unwilling listener, try to ignore your partner's words, just as you would any other distracting noise in the night. One sleep researcher found a simple, effective way of coping with his wife's nocturnal prattle: He simply asks her to shut up. She says, "Okay," rolls over and sleeps silently the rest of the night.

## WAKING IN THE NIGHT

Everyone wakes in the night, but usually so briefly that we don't remember ever having awakened. The key to getting back to sleep is not to arouse yourself any more than you already are. Don't get out of bed or turn on the light. As soon as you realize you're awake, tell yourself you'll be back asleep soon and use strategies from chapter

4 to return to sleep. If your muscles feel tense, choose sleep inducers that will relax them. If you start worrying about not sleeping, play a mind game to distract yourself.

If you consistently wake up in the night and can't get back to sleep, get out of bed and return only when drowsy. If you don't fall asleep quickly, leave the bed again. You can also consolidate your sleep by cutting back on the amount of time you spend in bed. Go to bed an hour or two later and get up at your usual time to increase your sleep efficiency. Once you're sleeping solidly, you can gradually increase your sleep time.

## TEETH-GRINDING (BRUXISM)

Millions of men, women, and children—as many as 21 percent of adults—gnash their teeth throughout the night. Although they may not realize that they're "bruxists," their dentists and bed partners are all too aware that their jaws are in motion.

Bruxism may well be a matter of both mind and mouth. Anxiety and stress play a role in some cases. In other individuals, the causes include missing, elongated, or poorly filled teeth as well as minor defects, such as rough cusp ends. For them, dental repair work can eliminate or reduce nighttime grinding. Some people whose upper and lower jaws don't meet well—a condition called malocclusion—also become bruxists. If untreated, teeth grinding can cause serious damage to the teeth, gums, and muscles of the mouth and jaw as well as pain and muscle and tooth sensitivity.

In addition to proper dental treatment, other approaches have helped teeth grinders sleep better. Hypnosis is one. While in a hypnotic trance, patients repeat the phrase, "Lips together, teeth apart," and visualize themselves sleeping peacefully with their jaws still. Biofeedback can also help sleepers become aware that they're moving their mouth and learn to stop.

One of the most effective treatments is a surprisingly simple exercise: Clench your teeth firmly for about five seconds. Relax for five. Repeat four to six times a day. In one study, after ten to twelve days of this self-treatment, 75 percent of the bruxists stopped grinding their teeth.

## LEG MOVEMENTS

Just as they're about to nod off, many sleepers feel a creeping sensation in their lower legs that's so uncomfortable they have to hop out of bed and walk until it stops. "Restless legs" is a common problem that may occur while sitting in a theater as well as while lying in bed. In mild cases, the discomfort passes quickly, but it can last for hours, forcing its victims to "wander like lost souls," as one sufferer put it, to relieve their aches.

Approximately one-third of the cases of restless legs are inherited. Others are linked to disease of the blood vessels, anemia, diabetes, spinal problems, polio, and poor circulation. Pregnant women are also susceptible. In one study, 11 percent of women experienced leg sensations in the second half of pregnancy. Sleep deprivation aggravates the problem, which often worsens with age.

Sleep researchers don't know what causes restless legs. Sleeping pills do *not* help; drugs that expand the blood vessels and improve circulation sometimes do. Caffeine may make the problem worse, perhaps by increasing nervous-system activity. One researcher found that young adults typically developed restless legs after drinking large amounts of coffee or cola. Iron, calcium, and vitamin E deficiencies may also trigger a problem.

Leg jerks that occur during the night—a condition called nocturnal myoclonus—can waken both sleepers and their bruised bed partners. Because the movements disrupt deep sleep, jerking legs may be responsible for 15 to 20 percent of complaints of insomnia. Even though each movement may last only five to fifteen seconds, a series may persist for several hours. Some patients' legs twitch every twenty to forty seconds.

Both men and women suffer from this problem, primarily when they're middle-aged or older. Various medical problems, including kidney disease, metabolic disorders, and sleep disorders such as apnea and narcolepsy, may play a role.

If your spouse complains about kicks in the night or your bed looks as if you've fought a battle with the sheets by morning, see your physician; he or she may perform neurological tests to rule out epilepsy or refer you to a sleep research center. Various drugs, including Valium (diazepam), a minor tranquilizer, and Clonopin (clonazepam), may help.

Leg cramping also bothers sleepers, particularly elderly ones. As they stretch their legs and feet during sleep, their muscles contract painfully. Neurologists Israel Weiner, M.D., and Henry Weiner, M.D., of Yale University believe that cramps occur when someone is asleep on his stomach or back and extends his foot, like a ballerina on her toes, while the muscles in his calf are relaxed. The result can be a sudden, uncontrollable contraction.

The easiest solution is to turn onto your side. If you invariably roll onto your back, keep the bed covers loose, prop them up to keep them off your feet, and rest your feet against a pillow to keep your toes from pointing. If you sleep on your stomach, let your feet dangle over the end of the bed. If you develop a cramp, grab your toes and force them toward your knees to bend the ankle and stretch out the cramped muscles in the back of the calf. You can also do a simple hamstring stretch before getting into bed to prevent problems: Stand about three feet from a wall and lean forward, keeping your heels on the floor. Hold this position for ten seconds, relax for four, and then repeat.

## NIGHT TERRORS

A "night terror" is the most intense form of anxiety you can experience. Victims wake up screaming, filled with an agonizing dread, their pupils dilated, perspiring heavily. Unresponsive and confused, they may not remember what frightened them, or they may recall only a single hallucination. While the attack lasts only seconds, victims may remain agitated and inconsolable for several minutes. Yet by morning they may forget they ever awoke.

Two-thirds of all adults report at least one such incident in their lives. Six percent experience one night terror a week; some wake up screaming two to four times a week. A third of children between ages three and eight may wake up because of night terrors. Males seem more vulnerable, usually experiencing their first attack between the ages of two and thirty. Most children outgrow night terrors by puberty, although boys, who mature later, experience them longer.

Like sleepwalking and bed-wetting, night terrors occur during partial arousal from deep sleep. Their cause is unknown. Two-thirds of night terrors occur in the first period of deep sleep within an hour to an hour and a half of falling asleep. The longer a sleeper spends in deep sleep, the more likely he is to have a night terror.

Night terrors aren't related to any particular personality or any form of mental disease, although fatigue and stress can trigger an attack. In one study, 33 percent of the patients said that their night terrors started at a time of major life change or trauma, such as losing a parent or being in an accident. About 75 percent felt that emotional stress intensified the problem. A high fever, head injuries, and trauma can also lead to attacks.

Researcher Ernest Hartmann, M.D., director of the sleep laboratory at Lemuel Shattuck Hospital in Boston, speculates that night terrors may be "a mild form of neurological disorder." Something in the brain—probably in the brainstem—may not have formed perfectly during maturation, so at certain times sudden arousal from deep sleep sets off an electrical discharge, rather like a minor epileptic seizure. The brain tracings of epileptics and night-terror victims are sometimes strikingly similar.

For some individuals, creating a sense of safety and security in their bedroom—by locking windows or leaving on a night-light—can help. In other cases, psychotherapy may help terrorized sleepers, particularly if they're bottling up negative feelings.

## NIGHTMARES

A nightmare is a bad dream that's more elaborate, more memorable, and far more unpleasant than other dreams. Unlike night terrors, nightmares occur in the second half of the night, during REM or dream sleep. Their victims recall at least fragments of their bad dreams, especially if they wake during the nightmare.

Nightmares may haunt sleepers as young as age two; the mean age for the onset of troubling dreams is 19.2 years. Three times as many women as men complain about nightmares, some reporting three terrifying dreams a week. If you have an occasional nightmare, consider it normal. You may have just as many—if not more— pleasant dreams, but you remember only the more troubling ones. You're also more likely to recall dreams during times of stress, exactly when your nighttime thoughts reflect the tensions of your days.

Various researchers have probed the personalities of nightmare sufferers, looking for clues to their troubled nights. Psychiatrist Ernest Hartmann, the leading expert on nightmares, found that individuals who had frequent nightmares all their lives were very open, not only to the outside world, but to their own impulses, wishes, and fears. He describes them as people with "thin boundaries": Their impulses, including normal hostile ones, get through their usual psychological defenses and invade their dreams. Their openness may make them vulnerable to mental illness or may lead them to artistic and creative achievements.

In his evaluation of thirty adults with chronic nightmares since childhood or adolescence, Anthony Kales, of Pennsylvania State University, found that they reported more frequent and intense dreams, which had more of an impact on their mood the next day. For 60 percent, major life crises preceded the onset of their nightmares; for 90 percent, stress increased their frequency.

Kales theorizes that nightmare sufferers, whom he describes as "distrustful, alienated, estranged, oversensitive, overreacting, and egocentric," may have difficulties dealing with interpersonal resentments. In their nightmares, they can discharge fears of hostility and extinguish unfinished anger and negative emotions. Yet expressing such emotions, even in a dream, provokes anxiety.

Fever, sleep deprivation, and withdrawal from drugs, including sleeping pills and alcohol, also increase nightmares. After taking drugs that suppress REM sleep, dream periods may rebound, lasting twice as long as usual. Dreams become more intense in these extended REM periods, which may explain why REM-rebound nightmares are especially bizarre and frightening.

If your nightmares seem to represent conflicts and problems in your waking life, you may want to seek professional counseling to resolve the problems causing your anxiety. Dreams have long been considered a path to the unconscious, and you may be able to learn more about yourself by exploring them. (Chapter 9 provides more information on putting your dreams—bad and good—to work for you.)

## PANIC ATTACKS

According to Peter Hauri, Ph.D., codirector of the sleep disorders center at Dartmouth University, people with panic attacks may suffer the same symptoms by night that they experience by day: a rapid heartbeat, sweaty palms, gasping for breath, and a feeling of disorientation and terror.

For three nights he compared the sleep patterns of fifteen panic patients with an equal number of normal sleepers and insomniacs. The panickers slept better than the insomniacs, about the same as normal sleepers. But during stage-2 sleep, which makes up about 60 percent of total sleep time, the panic sufferers showed signs of agitation, including increased eye movements, facial twitches, and rapid heart rate. Some actually woke up and had full-blown panic attacks.

In the past, many scientists believed that nighttime panic stemmed only from night terrors or nightmares. Hauri's findings offer further proof that panic attacks are a distinct problem that probably aren't triggered by psychological trouble but by a physiological disorder. Treatments include medication, relaxation, and behavioral approaches.

## HEARTBURN/GASTRIC REFLUX

Dozens of times in the night the middle-aged man would waken. His chest felt tight. There was a sour taste in his mouth. Sometimes he'd choke or cough violently. The problem: a backup of food and acid from the stomach into the esophagus.

According to William Orr, Ph.D., codirector of the Sleep Disorders Center at the Presbyterian Hospital in Oklahoma City, 7 percent of healthy adults report heartburn after meals every day; 36 percent, at least every week.

When stomach acids and enzymes back up into the esophagus by day, heartburn sufferers can swallow, belch, or quickly take an antacid. At night "recombinant refluxers," as Orr calls them, are at much greater risk. The noxious brew of stomach acids can pool in the esophagus for thirty minutes or longer, eroding the delicate lining and causing chronic inflammation. If the fluids are drawn into the lungs, they can lead to serious complications, including bronchitis, pneumonia, and pulmonary edema (a buildup of fluids in the lungs).

If you suffer from heartburn or belches by day or a burning, choking feeling by night, see your doctor. Various tests, including one with a portable twenty-four-hour monitor, can assess your ability to clear substances from your esophagus.

Elevating the head of your bed at night by putting six- to eight-inch blocks under the bedposts can prevent nighttime reflux. Also be sure not to lie down immediately after eating, to wear loose night clothing, and to avoid substances, such as caffeine and alcohol, that increase the production of stomach acids, or foods, such as citrus juices or vinegar, that can irritate the esophagus. Because obesity can cause or exacerbate this problem, try to slim down—for your stomach's and your sleep's sake. In serious cases, your doctor may also recommend antacids or drugs that aid clearance or lessen acid production.

# CHAPTER 7

# Rise and Shine: Overcoming Daytime Drowsiness

W e are a nation of sleepyheads. If you need proof, just look around: Chances are you'll catch someone midyawn. In all, 15 percent of the population may be chronically tired. Hypersomnia—excessive daytime sleepiness—drives more people to sleep disorders centers than any nocturnal malady.

Of 3,900 patients treated for sleep problems across the country over a two-year period, 51 percent complained most about sleepiness during the day. By comparison, 31 percent reported difficulties sleeping at night. Some daytime yawners had searched for help for ten to fifteen years. Yet many of the "waking wounded" don't relate their daytime daze to their nightime rest—or restlessness.

These sleepy people do manage to get by—barely. They're less alert, less amiable, less efficient than the well rested. They score lower on performance and intelligence tests; they make minor mistakes on the job. To others, they may seem lazy, rude, or dim-witted. When they take to the highways, they're downright dangerous, causing an estimated 20 percent of all accidents. If you're part of the drowsy crowd, this chapter will help you pinpoint what's wrong and tell you what you can do about it.

## WAKING UP IS HARD TO DO

Many different factors determine whether you bound out of bed or drag yourself wearily into the day. If you're dreaming when the alarm rings, you'll wake up more quickly than if you were in quiet sleep. The deeper your sleep stage at arousal, the longer it will take you to feel alert.

But waking up to full alertness and ability always takes time. One sleep researcher tested the hand grips of healthy college men during the day and upon arising. Their average strength was 13 percent below par on waking and took two minutes to return to normal. In sleep laboratories, volunteers who managed to silence a roaring alarm in a split second required at least thirty seconds to feel alert.

Bounding out of bed is always harder if you've been up several times in the night. A study at Henry Ford Hospital in Detroit found that the number and type of arousals in the night directly affect daytime sleepiness. The briefest, least disruptive arousals occurred during the lightest sleep stages.

If prying your eyelids open requires a supreme effort, start the day slowly. Develop a ritual to ease you into the day, just as you rely on one to soothe you into the night. Turn on the radio and listen to some music or news for a few minutes. Then wiggle your toes. Stretch your legs. Slowly work your way up your body until you lift your hands over your head and stretch from head to toe. Sit up, swinging your legs over the side of the bed. To get your blood circulating, bend forward at the waist, press your palms together and rub vigorously, pumping harder and harder for a few seconds. Lift your shoulders, as if you were shrugging them, hold briefly and release. Then stand up and face the day.

## ARE YOU WEARING YOURSELF OUT?

We may all inherit certain energy levels, so high-octane parents may well have lively offspring. But whatever your energy legacy, many other factors are more important in determining how you feel day by day. If you're out of shape, your body may be functioning so inefficiently that you're permanently pooped.

"The more active you are, the more work you can do with less effort," explains Mona Shangold, M.D., director of the Sports Gynecology Center at Georgetown University in Washington, D.C. "Aerobic exercise (swimming, cycling, jogging) increases your maximum oxygen uptake, so that you can take in, deliver, and use more oxygen. It also stimulates the production of chemicals such as brain peptides, which promote alertness, so that mental energy goes up too." To energize body and mind, pick an aerobic exercise you enjoy and do it for twenty to thirty minutes three or four times a week.

Too much exercise, like too little, can sap energy. That's what happened to exercise guru Jane Fonda when she combined her regular workout with daily runs and Nautilus routines. In *Jane Fonda's Workout Book,* she wrote, "I was so tired it was hard to get out of bed, and so depressed that I did not want to anyway." Avoid pushing yourself too hard, particularly if you're not accustomed to regular exercise.

While exercise can prime your body for peak efficiency, you still need adequate fuel to keep things running

# EIGHT ENERGIZING TIPS

- Check with your doctor to rule out possible medical problems and to find out if any medications may be affecting your energy level.
- Exercise for at least twenty to thirty minutes three or four days a week.
- Start the day with a high-octane breakfast that includes protein (eggs, meat, cottage cheese). If you're too rushed to sit down and eat, blend up a healthful shake (1 cup skim milk, 1 egg, and 1 banana or ½ cup berries).
- Don't skip meals. In addition to breakfast, lunch, and dinner, plan healthful snacks, such as fresh fruit, for midmorning and midafternoon.
- Establish good sleep habits. (See chapter 3 for guidance.)
- Set aside some time during the day for a "stress break," and use it for meditation, deep breathing, relaxation exercises, or yoga. If you can't free up a half hour or hour, take several ten-minute time-outs throughout the day.
- Tune in to your daily rhythms. If you're a morning-loving "lark" (see page 121), schedule your most demanding tasks for early in the day. If you're a natural night "owl," start slow and wait until your energy peaks in the afternoon before you tackle too much.
- Think through your priorities at work and at home. With them in mind, make lists of what must be done now and what can be put off. Recognize the real limitations on what you can do and delegate tasks as much as possible.

smoothly. If you're dieting and getting fewer than one thousand calories a day, you're basically running on empty. Diet pills that contain caffeine compound the problem by making you too jittery to rest.

It is possible to lose weight without losing energy. The best approach is to eat balanced low-fat meals. Complex carbohydrates, such as pasta, rice, potatoes, and whole-grain breads, are the best energy sources for physical activity. They help keep the level of sugar in your blood steady and provide your muscles with the energy they need for strenuous workouts.

If you start to slump between meals, be careful when choosing a snack to perk yourself up. A candy bar or brownie will provide a temporary lift, but your body reacts to such sugary treats by producing extra insulin to lower your blood sugar level. The result: You feel hungrier—and less energetic—than before. Caffeine can also work against you in the long run. Heavy coffee or cola drinkers build up a tolerance to caffeine, so they have to drink more to get a stimulating effect.

Some people turn to alcohol or drugs when their energy sags. But alcohol in any form is a depressant that slows down the normal processes of the central nervous system and the liver. It also has a direct effect on the muscles, so that you feel weaker after drinking.

Stimulating drugs, including cocaine and "uppers," such as amphetamines, can also backfire. After their initial energy "kick," they begin to wear off, and users feel sleepy. Tolerance gradually develops, and larger amounts are needed as pick-me-ups. Sleepiness is not the only negative effect. As they become dependent on drugs, many users of stimulants become irritable, lose weight, descend into deep depressions, and experience blackouts. If you've been using stimulants for a long time, seek professional help in breaking the habit. Quitting cold turkey can lead to a frightening seesaw from extreme daytime sleepiness to intense nighttime restlessness.

## THE LOWDOWN ON CHRONIC LOWS

Feelings of sluggishness aren't always the result of lack of exercise or bad habits. Sometimes fatigue is a symptom of a serious medical problem. For instance, iron-deficiency anemia, which occurs when red blood cells don't contain enough iron, is an energy-zapping disorder that affects about 5 percent of all menstruating women. Blood tests can detect the problem; daily iron supplements correct it.

Loss of energy may also be one of the symptoms of premenstrual syndrome (PMS), but many women experience a premenstrual energy slump even if they don't have PMS. The reason is the normal monthly surge in progesterone, the hormone that prepares the uterus for pregnancy, after ovulation. "In animals, progesterone can be used as an anesthetic because it has a sedative effect," notes Barbara Parry, M.D., assistant professor of psychiatry at the University of California, San Diego. "Some women seem to be very sensitive to it." Increased progesterone may explain why many women feel so tired early in pregnancy.

Because birth control pills contain varying amounts of progesterone, they can affect a woman's energy levels. Researchers at the University of Salford in Great Britain who studied women athletes found that birth control pills reduced their maximum oxygen capacity (their bodies' ability to use energizing oxygen) by as much as 11 percent.

Fatigue is one of the classic symptoms of fibrositis, a mysterious disorder of the musculoskeletal system that singles out women in the prime of life as its victims. Symptoms include a flulike feeling, aches, pains, stiffness, and extreme tiredness. For years, doctors could find nothing wrong with the women who came to see them with these vague complaints. Sleep specialists revealed an unexpected common denominator: very light sleep.

"I believe fibrositis is a very common problem," says Harvey Moldofsky, M.D., professor of psychiatry and medicine at the University of Toronto. "And the cause seems to be the lack of restorative sleep." His prescription: developing good sleep habits and aerobic exercise, particularly swimming. "It helps build up energy and tolerance for discomfort," he says. In severe cases, small doses of tricyclic antidepressants may help.

Infectious diseases—colds, flus, urinary tract infections—are also energy busters. Some, such as mononucleosis (the "kissing disease" that causes fatigue, swelling of the lymph nodes under the jaw, fever, headache, and sore throat), can leave victims feeling exhausted for months.

Among the medical disorders that can cause sleepiness during the day as well as sleeplessness by night are extreme obesity, hypoglycemia (commonly called low blood sugar), hypothyroidism (too little thyroid hormone), diabetes, multiple sclerosis, and injuries to the brain and nervous system.

Many common medications, including antihistamines, allergy drugs, and antibiotics such as tetracycline, can cause drowsiness as a side effect. Painkilling drugs and sedatives can also be culprits. If you've been relying on sleeping pills to rest better at night, you may be feeling their residual effects during the day. Check with your doctor to see if any medications you're taking may be undermining your energy. Also be wary of alcohol, which can enhance the sleep-inducing effects of drugs.

## IS FATIGUE ALL IN YOUR HEAD?

If you waken by dawn's earliest light long before you want to get out of bed, the reason may be depression, a common problem that affects the nights and days of millions of men and women. While depressed people often feel sad, a clinical depression is far more than the blues. Depressed individuals may feel anxious and agitated, lack energy, be unable to function normally, and withdraw from others. Virtually all have sleep problems, particularly early wakenings.

Sometimes depression follows a life crisis, such as a death in the family; often it sneaks up on its victims, striking without any apparent reason. "You can be depressed without knowing what you're experiencing," says psychiatrist Susan Fiester, M.D., associate medical director of Nashua Brookside Hospital in New Hampshire. "You may not feel sad, but you may lose your motivation, you can't sleep or eat, and you don't have any energy." Among depression's other symptoms are

- Loss of appetite and weight
- Loss of sexual desire
- Neglect of appearance and hygiene
- Heart "palpitations" or flutters
- Shortness of breath
- Impaired memory
- Inability to concentrate
- Indecisiveness
- Illogical thinking
- Feelings of guilt
- Isolation from others

Some people, especially teenagers, sleep more when they're depressed. Most adults sleep less. As their depression becomes worse, they get less total sleep and less deep sleep and have more periods of wakefulness in the night.

Depression dramatically changes sleep stages. Normally, the first REM or dream period begins ninety minutes after bedtime and is relatively brief, with REM periods becoming longer during the second half of the night. Individuals with certain types of depression enter REM within an hour of falling asleep. Just when most people are beginning their longest dreams of the night, they've completed REM. They wake up, unable to fall back to sleep.

Like any problem underlying disturbed sleep, depression must be treated before sleep can improve. Treatments that work for insomnia, such as sleep restriction or relaxation exercises, provide no lasting relief. The use of sleeping pills is especially hazardous because some can be a means of suicide, which is always a danger in depression.

Without treatment, depression can trap its victims in a black cocoon of misery for months, even a year. The choice of treatment depends on the type and severity of the depression. Exercise lifts mild depressions. Psychotherapy helps improve the patients' relationships and social interactions. Antidepressant medications correct an imbalance of chemicals within the brain. Daily exposure to very bright light helps those with Seasonal Affective Disorder, who become depressed in the dark days of winter.

Other emotional problems can also take a toll on your energy. The "nervous energy" that propels some people into seemingly perpetual motion is often nerve-fraying anxiety. Eventually it generates so much tension that it saps internal resources, and its victims run out of steam.

Not dealing with emotional issues also burns up psychic energy. "Some people stay so busy they're too tired to face up to a real problem," says Jean Hamilton, M.D., a psychiatrist in Washington, D.C. "Fatigue becomes a way of avoiding a difficult situation." Your best bet is to step back and pinpoint your problems and then tackle each one individually—with professional help, if necessary.

## SLEEP APNEA

The most common reason for sleepiness is not enough sleep. But what may matter more than total hours in bed is the number of arousals in the night. "In the last ten years, we've been seeing more and more patients who can sleep for eight to eighteen hours yet still feel sleepy during the day," says Michael Bonnet, M.D., director of the sleep laboratory at the Loma Linda Veterans Administration Medical Center. "Their sleep isn't working. It's interrupted sometimes as often as once every minute."

The primary culprit: sleep apnea. Translated from the Greek words meaning "no" and "breath," sleep apnea is exactly that: the absence of breathing for a brief period. Victims have at least thirty such episodes, each lasting fifteen to sixty seconds, every night. Some stop breathing as often as four hundred to five hundred times before morning. According to recent estimates, three million Americans, including 60 percent of men over fifty, may have apnea. In this group men outnumber women by thirty to one.

The first clue to this problem is the sound of the sleeper. Apneics raise such a ruckus that they drown out other snorers. In most cases, an obstruction in the airway, such as flabby throat muscles or a large tongue, blocks the flow of air to the lungs. The brain, signaled that the body needs oxygen, rouses the sleeper, not quite to the point of awakening, but just enough so that he sucks in air loudly and vigorously. As he struggles to breathe, he may flail his arms and legs, snort, choke, and gasp.

Obesity greatly increases the risk of obstructive sleep apnea. Other common causes are ear, nose, and throat disorders, such as large tonsils and adenoids; an abnormal upper airway; neurological diseases (polio, myasthenia

# SIGNS OF SLEEP APNEA

Obesity
Excessive daytime sleepiness
Insomnia
Heavy snoring
Abnormal activity during sleep
Morning headaches
Intellectual and personality changes
Depression
Impotence
Bed-wetting
Hypertension
Irregular heartbeats during sleep

gravis, and so on); pulmonary disease; and heart disorders. In children, large tonsils and adenoids may cause apnea by night and impulsiveness, aggressiveness, and other bad behaviors by day.

At any age, apnea devastates daytime functioning. Apneics fall asleep in their seats and on their feet, even while eating, driving, or making love. Long naps, also interrupted by breath stoppages, make them feel groggier rather than more alert.

Because chronically low levels of oxygen can affect the heart and lungs, apnea can threaten life as well as destroy its quality. Its victims often develop headaches, increased irritability, aggressiveness, impotence, and other sexual problems. In his studies, psychiatrist Anthony Kales, M.D., of Pennsylvania State University School of Medicine in Hershey, found that severe apnea led to impairments in thinking, perception, memory, communication, and ability to learn new information.

The last few years have brought dramatic new treatments for this debilitating problem. The simplest is a matter of position: By lying on their sides instead of their backs, individuals with apnea can drastically reduce the number of times they stop breathing in the night. In 1985, Rosalind Cartwright, Ph.D., director of the Sleep Disorders Center of Rush-Presbyterian-Saint Luke's Medical Center in Chicago, reported twice as many breath stoppages in patients who rest on their backs rather than their sides, possibly because their tongues fall backward over the airway.

To teach them to sleep on their sides, Cartwright placed a gravity-sensitive monitor on the chests of ten men with apnea. If they lay on their backs for more than fifteen seconds, an auditory signal roused them. The device worked, decreasing the number of times they stopped breathing in the night. A pillow attached around the waist with a belt can have the same effect.

Another smart strategy for apneics is losing weight. A study at Johns Hopkins University in Baltimore found that moderate weight loss dramatically reduces breath stoppages during sleep. When fifteen overweight men with moderate-to-severe apnea lost an average of twenty pounds each, they had fewer apneic episodes, slept better, and felt more awake during the day. In fact, their sleep improved as much as that of patients who'd lost much more weight after undergoing surgery to bypass their intestines.

A new medical treatment is Continuous Positive Airway Pressure (CPAP). Each night sleepers place small masks or prongs over their noses. These are hooked up to a machine on the bedside table, which pushes a continuous supply of oxygen—sometimes heated and humidified—directly into the upper throat. This tiny bit of air pressure opens up the airway and seems to increase muscle tone. In one study by David Rapoport, M.D., of New York University Medical Center, CPAP totally eliminated the apneas of thirty-eight hospitalized patients who'd been experiencing 27 to 120 breath stoppages per hour.

If other treatments fail, surgery can provide hope. In the past, surgeons created a permanent opening in the windpipe—a tracheostomy—for air to enter. But the procedure can be dangerous and difficult, because apneics often have short, thick necks that require special techniques and tubing. While tracheostomy does lessen daytime sleepiness and improve performance, about 30 percent of patients who undergo the surgery stop using the tracheostomy because of irritation and other complications.

A newer procedure, called uvulo-palato-pharyngoplasty, literally resculpts the upper airway by removing the tonsils and soft tissue of the throat. At six American medical centers, about half of 314 patients who'd had this operation had a 50 percent reduction in apneas (from sixty-five per hour to an average of forty-five per hour) one to nine months later. An added benefit is that the surgery usually eliminates snoring. "About 90 percent of patients don't snore afterward," says Wallace Mendelson, M.D., of the National Institute of Mental Health. "But this is major surgery and a lot to go through simply to stop snoring."

## NARCOLEPSY

The forty-one-year-old fireman couldn't remember a time in his life when he didn't feel sleepy. Even though he often napped during the day, he couldn't stay awake when he went out with his wife in the evening. Any expression of emotion—from laughing at a joke to the excitement of a fire—made him extremely weak, sometimes jeopardizing his own safety and that of his comrades. For years, he wondered what was wrong. Finally, a sleep disorders center provided the answer: narcolepsy.

Narcolepsy is a mysterious disorder of sudden, irresistible sleep attacks that occur throughout the day, often at times of intense emotion. Regardless of how much they sleep at night, narcoleptics cannot keep their eyes open during the day. They become sleepy, not just during quiet activities, such as reading and watching television, but while driving or talking to friends. While narcolepsy affects two hundred thousand Americans, only a third of the nation's narcoleptics know what's wrong with them. Many spend more than a decade searching for help before their problem is correctly diagnosed.

Narcolepsy has a wide range of symptoms. Some narcoleptics slump into sleep several times during the day. Others continue to do routine tasks, like drying dishes or driving, even though they've fallen asleep. They may waken only after cutting themselves with the blade of a knife or driving off the side of the road.

As their symptoms worsen, narcoleptics may wake often at night, craving sweets or other food. Sometimes they develop sleep apnea. During the transitions from wakefulness to sleep and back again, they often experience realistic, horrible sensations and hallucinations, such as snakes crawling over them. When they wake up, they may be unable to move for several minutes because of a condition called sleep paralysis.

Many narcoleptics also suffer from cataplexy, a partial or complete weakening of muscle tone, usually triggered by excitement or intense emotion. One woman became weak whenever she began to scold or spank her child; a stockbroker would lose all muscle tone while negotiating a big trade. Usually narcoleptics remain conscious of words and sounds during a cataplectic attack, but may not remember the details of what happened.

Sleep researchers do not know the specific cause of narcolepsy, but they believe that a disorder of the sleep-wake mechanism interferes with both daytime wakefulness and nighttime sleep. Narcolepsy is hereditary, and there is a one-in-twenty chance that the children of a narcoleptic parent will develop the problem. Psychological difficulties are common in narcoleptics, but they seem to be the result, not the cause, of the illness.

Narcolepsy is diagnosed on the basis of four classic symptoms:

- Irresistible daytime sleep attacks
- Cataplexy (muscle weakness)
- Sleep paralysis
- Hallucinations while falling asleep or waking up


Treatment depends on the severity of the problem. Those with mild to moderate symptoms may be able to cope by maintaining good sleep habits, such as keeping regular bedtimes, and getting frequent daytime naps. For more severe cases, physicians can prescribe various medications, including stimulants to overcome daytime sleepiness, antidepressants, and drugs to prevent muscle weakness. For further information, contact the American Narcolepsy Association, Post Office Box 5846, Stanford, California 94304.


## SLEEP DRUNKENNESS

Remember the worst Monday morning of your life, when you slept through the alarm and pulled yourself out of bed feeling disoriented and confused? That's how people with sleep drunkenness feel every morning, regardless of how much or how well they slept the night before. Sleep "drunks" can barely manage to get themselves ready for the day, stumbling as they walk and ignoring a whistling kettle of boiling water or the toast burning in the oven. Their profound confusion, disorientation, and lack of coordination may last from fifteen minutes to up to four hours. As the day wears on, they gradually start to feel better.

Sleep drunkenness is relatively rare. Its victims usually fall asleep within minutes of going to bed and have normal sleep stages. If given the chance, they'd sleep from 9:00 P.M. to 2:00 P.M. the following afternoon. Most feel drowsy in the day and also suffer depression, headaches, poor concentration, mood swings, and anxiety. Sleep deprivation, exhausting physical activity, and the use of sleeping pills may aggravate the problems. If you suspect that you have this problem, check with your doctor or a sleep disorders center.

## PERIODIC PROBLEMS

Sometimes excessive daytime sleepiness waxes and wanes over several weeks or months. If you feel that you're going through cycles of extreme drowsiness, keep a sleep diary so that you can identify the times of greatest sleepiness. One such problem is the Klein-Levin Syndrome, a disorder of certain control centers in the brain that occurs most often in teenage boys. They experience sleep "binges" and may also become irritable, confused, voraciously hungry, and sexually uninhibited. They usually outgrow all these symptoms by age forty.

# CHAPTER 8

# Resetting Your Biological Clock

W e've all got rhythms—in the flow of our hormones, the division of our cells, the sensitivity of our taste buds, the sharpness of our memories. Most of the time, we're unaware of these cycles, but one rhythm—sleeping and waking—is too obvious and too important for any of us to ignore.

Some common sleep problems are really rhythm disturbances, often caused by the demands of our high-speed, nonstop world. If you have a problem falling asleep too late or too early or if you have to contend with jet lag or changing work shifts, this chapter can help you get your rhythms back into sync with the world around you.

## ARE YOU A NIGHT OWL?

"I understand why they execute condemned men at dawn," Pablo Picasso once quipped. "I just have to see the dawn in order to have my head roll all by itself." In all likelihood, the artist was a night owl, and like others of the breed, he loathed the hours of the early morning. By comparison, "larks" rise as brightly as the sun.

There is a subtle but profound difference between larks and owls: The larks' body temperatures peak early in the day, while night owls require more time, not only to wake up but to warm up. Their body temperatures may not reach their maximum until early evening. If they try to go to sleep at a normal bedtime, they find it impossible to drift off. After hours of thrashing and turning, they finally fall asleep at 3:00 or 4:00 A.M. The following morning they may sleep through even the loudest of alarms.

While he was a student at Stanford University, sleep researcher Charles Czeisler, M.D., turned into a night owl after commuting frequently from coast to coast. To reset his body clock, he "rewound" it: He gradually moved his bedtime back, tinkering with his internal rhythms until they were in phase with the schedule he wanted to keep. This approach, called chronotherapy, has helped many others with the same difficulty: delayed sleep-phase syndrome.

If you lie awake for hours in the night and have difficulty getting out of bed in the morning, you may have this clockworks problem. Maybe it began in childhood, when you snuck a flashlight beneath the covers so that you could read into the night. Or an accident, a late-night job, or an illness may have forced you to stay up late. Once your body became accustomed to late nights, it insisted on sticking to this new schedule.

As long as night owls can sleep late yet manage to work and spend time with family and friends, they can be completely content. But if you have to conform to a nine-to-five routine, you're almost certain to have problems—in bed and out.

---

# STAYING IN RHYTHM

- Don't nap in the daytime.
- Go to bed only when you're sleepy.
- Wake up at the same time every day, including weekends.
- Schedule your most productive hours for the same time every day.
- Establish a daily routine for work, exercise, relaxation, meals, and sleep. Stick to it as closely as possible.

---

The standard solutions for insomnia—relaxation therapies, sleep restriction, cognitive focusing—won't help. You have to reset your biological clock. It's impossible for night owls to go to bed earlier and "phase-advance" their sleep time. But you can "phase-delay" your sleep time, shifting your bedtime later and later until you move it around the clock to a reasonable hour.

Here's how phase-delay chronotherapy works: If you normally fall asleep at 3:00 A.M., you move your bedtime back by three hours. For three or four days, you force yourself to stay up later and go to bed at 6:00 A.M., sleeping for your normal length of time. Then you shift your bedtime to 9:00 A.M. After a few more days, you start going to bed at noon. By the end of a two-week period, you'll be getting into bed at midnight and sleeping through the night.

Chronotherapy is not easy. On some days, you may be going to bed when everyone else is eating breakfast or lunch. To survive this topsy-turvy schedule, you need lots of support and a place where you can sleep comfortably at any time of the day. Some people end up staying in a hospital or sleep center during the entire time.

A new alternative to chronotherapy is light exposure. If you spend time outdoors or under very bright indoor lights in the morning and stay away from light in the evening, you can cue your body to advance your sleep cycles and let you fall asleep earlier.

## TOO EARLY TO BED

Some people, usually older ones, develop the opposite problem: They become irresistibly sleepy early in the evening and wake up in the middle of the night, ready to start a new day. "A lot of elderly people say they can't stay up late anymore or that they're up with the dawn," says Harvey Moldofsky, M.D., of the University of Toronto. "They may well have mild cases of advanced sleep-phase disorder."

One of Moldofsky's patients, a sixty-two-year-old man who had gone to work before dawn for thirty years, sought help after he retired. Each evening he'd become so sleepy by 6:30 P.M. that he'd nod off while eating, talking, reading, watching TV, even riding his bicycle or driving. At 3:00 A.M., he'd wake up feeling full of energy and jog in the dark for an hour.

To reset this man's clock, Moldofsky had him go to bed earlier than usual: Over a two-week period, he advanced his bedtime by three hours every two days, so that he went to bed at 3:30 P.M., then 12:30 P.M., then 9:30 A.M. Eventually he worked his way around the clock, and settled into a schedule of going to bed at 11:00 P.M. and rising at 6:00 A.M.

## JET LAG

Jet lag is the price our Stone Age bodies pay for living in a Space Age world. While we can travel across time zones in hours, resetting our watches with a flick of the fingers, our bodies and minds need much more time to adjust. In fact, for each time zone you cross, you need a day to adapt.

Jet lag refers to the period of adjustment when you're temporarily off-cue. Its symptoms include fatigue, lapses of attention, cloudy vision, short-term memory loss, digestive problems, and erratic sleep-wake cycles. They persist until the rhythms of the hormones and chemical signals that orchestrate body functions are restored.

If you arrive in London on a flight from New York, Big Ben may be tolling its bells for 9:00 A.M., but your body clock insists that it's only 4:00 A.M. That night your sleep stages are altered, with REM sleep appearing later and not lasting as long as usual. A more normal sleep pattern appears on the second night, although sleep still tends to be fragmented and brief.

For about five days, you may wake up at dawn unable to return to sleep. Your body temperature rhythms may not become synchronized with the new schedule for a week. The older you are, the harder you'll find the adjustment. Traveling east to west creates fewer problems, perhaps because it's easier to push your clock backward than forward.

Some degree of jet lag seems inevitable, but researchers have found new ways to minimize its impact. One is by exposure to bright white light. Alfred Lewy, M.D., Ph.D., director of the Sleep and Mood Disorders Laboratory of the Oregon Health Sciences University in Portland, has found that carefully timed light exposure can prepare us for trips across continents or oceans.

# BEATING JET LAG

- Begin the time shift before you leave home. If you're heading for Europe or Australia, set one clock in your house to the time zone of your destination. Gradually begin going to bed and getting up earlier if you're traveling east, and staying up and getting up later if you're heading west.
- Leave home rested and relaxed. Try to avoid last-minute hassles, such as frantic packing the night before your trip and a mad rush to the airport.
- Dress in loose, comfortable clothes for the trip. Take your shoes off on the flight. Don't try to work en route.
- Stretch often. Get up and stroll around the plane. Alternately tense and relax different muscle groups as you sit.
- Travel with a friend if possible. Companionship eases the tedium of long flights.
- Eat lightly during the flight.
- Drink little, if any, alcohol. You don't want to add a hangover to your jet lag problems.
- Don't smoke. Cigarettes irritate your eyes, ears, and throat in the zero-humidity of a plane.
- Instead of coffee, tea, or cola, stick with water or fruit juices.
- Schedule your arrival late in the day so that you can go to bed as soon as possible but still stay in sync with your new time zone.
- On a short trip, stay on your home time, eating and sleeping when you normally would.
- On a long trip, start living by your new time frame immediately. When in Rome, eat, sleep, work, and rest when the Romans do.
- Stop for a day or two of rest if you're traveling halfway around the world.

- Rely on familiar sleep rituals or relaxation exercises to ease you into sleep.
- Plan a quiet, relaxed schedule for the first two or three days of your trip.

"Light early in the day seems to shift the body's inner clock to an earlier time," he says. "Light late in the day seems to shift the clock later." Even if the day is cloudy, outdoor light is bright enough to have an effect. To get the same results with indoor lighting, you need special lights four times as bright as ordinary incandescent bulbs.

If you're traveling from the West to the East Coast, across three time zones, Lewy recommends going outdoors in the morning before you leave to advance your biological rhythms. If you're going west, spend time outdoors in the late afternoon or evening. For a much longer trip, such as a flight from the West Coast to Europe, he advises that you avoid sunlight before 10:00 A.M. but seek it afterward. (See box.)

Certain foods also influence the brain chemicals that affect alertness. Proteins, such as meat and eggs, stimulate substances that perk us up, such as epinephrine (adrenaline). Carbohydrates such as pasta or rice boost production of serotonin, a neurotransmitter that ushers in the sleep phase of our cycles. In addition, according to Charles Ehret, Ph.D., a biologist at the Argonne National Laboratory in Illinois, fasting makes people more receptive to the introduction of a new cycle, probably because it influences the body's natural pattern of energy reserves, such as sugar stores in the liver.

Using these insights into food and mood, Ehret has devised a strategy for minimizing jet lag. Here's how it would work if you were leaving on a 9:30 P.M. Wednesday flight from Chicago to Paris:

1. Sunday, three days prior to departure: A feast day. Eat eggs or meat for protein at breakfast. Also load up on proteins at lunch, but have a high-carbohydrate dinner, such as pasta.
2. Monday: Fast day. Eat lightly, having foods like fruit and yogurt.
3. Tuesday, day before departure: Repeat the feast pattern with a bacon-and-egg breakfast, meaty lunch, and dinner of pasta, beans, or potatoes (all carbohydrates).
4. Wednesday: Eat lightly. Drink no coffee or tea until 6:00 P.M. From then until midnight Chicago time, drink several cups of strong tea or coffee.
5. On board, turn out lights. Forget the movie. Avoid conversation, and try to nap. Ask the flight attendant to hold your dinner until shortly before arrival (close to Parisian breakfast time). Before landing, get up, turn on the lights, stretch, walk around, breathe deeply, clap hands, or talk.
6. On arrival, have a protein-rich lunch. Don't nap. Do light exercises and deep breathing. Put off sleep until late evening.

Another way to cushion jet lag's jolt is to use L-tryptophan, a natural sleep-inducer (see page 74), to help you fall asleep at your new bedtime. In an experiment with Marines airlifted over seven time zones to Okinawa, Cheryl Spinwebber, of the Naval Health Research Center in San Diego, found that two to four grams of tryptophan, taken en route and on the first three nights in Japan, increased average sleep times by fifty-two minutes. "That's almost an hour of good rest," she says, "so we're talking about a big piece of sleep."

The box on page 125 outlines other commonsense guidelines for avoiding jet lag.

# HOW TO BEAT JET LAG

Traveling West (to Earlier Time Zone)

| Time Difference | Get Outdoor Light From |
|---|---|
| 2 hours | 4:00 P.M. to 6:00 P.M.* |
| 4 hours | 2:00 P.M. to 6:00 P.M. |
| 6 hours plus | 12:00 P.M. to 6:00 P.M. |

Traveling East (to Later Time Zone)

| Time Difference | Stay Indoors From | Get Outdoor Light From |
|---|---|---|
| 2 hours | | 6:00 A.M.* to 8:00 A.M. |
| 4 hours | | 6:00 A.M. to 10:00 A.M. |
| 6 hours | | 6:00 A.M. to 12:00 P.M. |
| 8 hours | 6:00 A.M. to 8:00 A.M. | 8:00 A.M. to 2:00 P.M. |
| 10 hours | 6:00 A.M. to 10:00 A.M. | 10:00 A.M. to 4:00 P.M. |

* This table assumes that the sun will rise at 6:00 A.M. and set at 6:00 P.M. in the new time zone. If it doesn't, readjust the times in the table to reflect actual times.

# SHIFTING GEARS

Changes in your sleeping and eating patterns may ease your transition from one work shift to another. Biologist Charles Ehret, of Argonne National Laboratory, who has studied natural rhythms for more than thirty-five years, developed these guidelines for workers shifting from the day shift on Friday (8:00 A.M. to 4:00 P.M.) to the afternoon shift on Monday (4:00 P.M. to midnight):

- Sleep late on Saturday and eat sparingly all day, choosing soups, salads, fruits. Avoid carbohydrates such as pasta.
- Sleep late Sunday. Eat a big, high-protein meal about 3:00 P.M. (breakfast time on Monday) and have a high-protein meal about 8:00 P.M. (Monday's lunch time).
- Eat a big high-carbohydrate supper about 2:00 A.M. Monday. Go to bed around 7:00 A.M.

## SHIFT WORK

About 20 percent of Americans work the night or evening shifts or rotate between daytime and nighttime hours. Trying to "beat the clock," they end up being beaten by it. Shift workers get less sleep than others, averaging only 5.6 hours per night, and often feel tired and edgy when they wake up.

The "graveyard" shift, from midnight to 8:00 A.M., takes the greatest toll. Even after years of nightwork, many employees never really adjust. Performance and efficiency are notoriously lower among night laborers. Meter readers make more errors at night; steel workers have slower reaction times; phone operators take longer to answer incoming calls.

As body temperature and alertness drop, we all make small but serious errors, thinking "right" but turning left, pushing the "up" button when we want to go down, misreading simple instructions or maps. The miscalculations that led to the most serious mishap in the history of U.S. nuclear energy—at Three Mile Island in Pennsylvania in 1980—were made at 4:00 A.M. by workers who'd been changing shifts every week.

The problem with frequent shift changes is that the body needs three or four weeks to settle into a new routine. Unable to adapt to a new time frame every week, many workers try to live two lives—as night people during the work week and day people on weekends.

The stress of these efforts shows up in frequent reports of digestive problems, marital upsets, and emotional disruptions. Shift workers are twice as likely as day workers to report trouble sleeping. When Richard Coleman, Ph.D., a clinical instructor in psychiatry at Stanford University, surveyed 1,500 factory and production shift workers at thirteen plants in the United States, he found that the rotating shift workers were less satisfied with their jobs than the day workers.

At one plant, the workers' changing schedules had the same impact as traveling around the world every twenty days. Not surprisingly, 76 percent did not sleep well. To compensate, they napped more, drank more coffee (five to ten cups a day), used over-the-counter stimulants, drank more alcohol, and took more sleeping pills. In one study, 67 percent of shift workers used alcohol at bedtime at least once a week, while 12 percent took sleeping pills. The majority said they were most alert on their time off and least alert during work hours. About 50 percent admitted falling asleep on the job at least once a week; 15

percent reported falling asleep while driving to and from work at least once in the previous three months.

According to the National Center for Health Statistics, in Hyattsville, Maryland, 27 percent of men and 16 percent of women on changing schedules rotate in the "wrong" direction, that is, opposing the natural tendencies of the body's internal circadian clocks. Usually they "phase-advance" by eight hours, so that workers go from days to nights to evenings. Yet the opposite type of rotation— from days to evenings to nights—fosters greater satisfaction and productivity.

Careful planning before a shift change also helps. Coleman advises that you anticipate a new shift by gradually changing the hours you sleep on the days between your old and new shifts. Short-acting sleeping pills can also help for a night or two when your schedule changes.

Here are some other guidelines for smoothing a change in shifts:

- Eat meals at the same time every day, including days off.
- Try to sleep at least four hours during the same time every day. It's better to aim for one long sleep stint rather than two shorter ones. However, if you work nights and usually go to sleep at 8:00 A.M., you may want to do the same on Saturday and Sunday but wake up at noon so that you can spend time with your family or friends.
- When you try to sleep during the day, darken the room with heavy draperies.
- Block out daytime noise with earplugs, music, or the hum of an air conditioner or fan.
- Try to exercise daily, scheduling workouts after sleep rather than before. Stick to the same times on your days off.

- Avoid or cut down on coffee and other caffeine-containing substances.
- Stay away from stimulating activities, such as watching an exciting sports event, before your bedtime.
- Eat high-protein meals before work and high-carbohydrate meals before sleep. Avoid going to bed feeling hungry or full.
- Don't smoke for several hours before your bedtime.
- When you get home, take time to unwind and relax before getting into bed.
- Don't drink alcoholic beverages to get to sleep.
- Don't try to shift gears by changing your schedule on weekends or days off. Your body will be more confused by the erratic time changes than it was when you changed shifts.
- Involve the entire family. Shift work takes a toll on everyone in the home. Your spouse and children may resent your absence at night and your insistence on quiet by day. Talk about these issues and enlist their help in finding ways and times to spend a few hours together each day.

# CHAPTER 9

# The Late Show: Tuning In to Your Dreams

We soar above the earth, tumble through space, dash naked down city streets, visit alien worlds where animals talk and trees are blue. When we dream, we enter the realm of the impossible, the improbable, and the absurd. And when we wake up—sometimes with our hearts pounding in fear, sometimes chuckling over a joke we've already forgotten—we wonder what it all means.

Dreams have fascinated and baffled men and women for centuries. The ancient Egyptians believed they were messages from the gods; the Chinese saw them as voyages into the realm of ghosts and spirits. Early in this century, Sigmund Freud, the father of psychoanalysis, argued that dreams are "the royal road to the unconscious," crammed with symbols and laden with psychological significance.

The very fact that we spend two hours a night and five to six years of our lives dreaming indicates how crucial dreams must be. In fact, our brains seem to crave them.

When volunteers in sleep labs were awakened throughout the night so that they couldn't dream, they altered their normal sleep patterns the following night so that they'd start dreaming earlier and dream for longer periods.

The most obvious sign that you're dreaming is the back-and-forth motion of your eyes beneath closed lids. During the four or five periods of Rapid Eye Movement, or REM, sleep during the night, the muscles of your arms, legs, and trunk are paralyzed, while your fingers and toes may twitch. Your temperature, heart rate, and blood pressure rise. Your breathing pattern changes, as does the flow of hormones and other crucial chemicals through your bloodstream. Whether male or female, you show signs of sexual arousal. The tiny muscles of your middle ear vibrate. Your brain is as active as it is during waking hours. And as you dream, you "see" without opening your eyes, "hear" without listening to a sound in the room, "feel" without touching.

You dream every night, and the plot of your dreams follows a definite pattern, much like that of an old-time movie serial or a made-for-television miniseries. The opening segment, which occurs about ninety minutes after you fall asleep and lasts for ten or fifteen minutes, introduces the main characters. The next two or three segments consist of flashbacks, flashforwards, and restatements of the central theme.

The plot culminates in the last and longest dream of the night, just before dawn. This is the dream you're most likely to recall—and to be mystified by. Making sense of it can be as difficult as figuring out what's happening in the last scene of an opera if you've missed the previous acts.

But dreams can be deciphered—and not just by experts. Through books, seminars, informal networks, or dream discussion groups, thousands of ordinary dreamers are paying close attention to the stories they tell themselves as they sleep. This chapter explains why and shows how you, too, can remember your dreams and put them to work for you.

## THE MEANING OF DREAMS

According to classic Freudian theory, a dream event actually expresses a submerged wish or fear. A dream of falling, for instance, symbolizes fear of loss of love, which might stem from childhood anxiety and anger toward a mother who was frustratingly remote. Therapists trained in other analytic perspectives might contend that the fall represents a declining career or succumbing to a romantic or erotic temptation. Yet all would agree that the fall represents something important in the dreamer's unconscious.

But a new breed of dream scientists has questioned whether our dreams—good, bad, or bizarre—really mean anything at all. These researchers contend that dreams are the products, not of buried impulses, but of the brain's routine nighttime activity.

According to psychiatrists Robert McCarley and J. Allan Hobson, of the Massachusetts Mental Health Center in Boston, certain cells in the brainstem are jostled by normal electrical activity during REM sleep and send random messages to the regions of the brain that control vision, hearing, and movement. Registering the fact that cells usually involved in movement or perception are turned on, the higher brain flips through scenes and characters stored in its memory and fits them together into a plausible scenario, or explanation, which we experience as a dream.

Are dreams no more than a matter of cells bumping into each other in the night? Or are they tunnels into hidden recesses of the psyche? The debate is far from

## A THOUSAND DREAMERS

Here is how one thousand readers of *Psychology Today* responded to a survey on dreams:

• Ninety-five percent said they remember at least some of their dreams.
• Sixty-eight percent have a recurring dream. The most common is being chased or falling, followed by returning to a childhood home, flying, appearing naked or scantily clad in public, and being unprepared for an exam.
• Thirty-eight percent can control the course of their dreams.
• Twenty-eight percent had died in their dreams. (According to the experts, this isn't as ominous as it sounds, for the "death" may represent giving up some negative part of their personalities.)
• Forty-five percent dream about celebrities, including Tom Selleck, Michael Jackson, Elvis Presley, Bob Hope, Johnny Carson, the pope, and the president.

over, but the views of the mind analysts and the brain researchers are not as contradictory as they may initially seem. In the last decade, both groups have contributed many tiny pieces to the puzzle of what dreaming really is. Taken as a whole, their findings suggest that our dreams aren't purely psychological or entirely physiological, but creations of both our busy brains and our unconscious minds.

## THE NIGHT SHIFT

As a biological process, dreaming is indeed predictable, rhythmic, and necessary, not unlike digestion—although in dreams, images and ideas, not snacks and suppers, are broken down and processed. In fact, we have more dreams than meals in our lives: 1,825 dreams a year, or 127,750 by the time we reach age seventy.

One controversial theory about dreaming contends that we're better off forgetting our dreams. According to biologist Francis Crick, Ph.D., who won a Nobel Prize for his work in deciphering DNA, our basic genetic blueprint, dreaming may be a process of systematic "unlearning." As he explains it, brain cells, or neurons, fire electrical signals in response to different stimuli, such as sights or sounds. Bombarded by such inputs during the day, networks of neurons become overloaded and connect different memories in different ways—some correct and legitimate, some nonsensical. During the night, our dreams reinforce the correct associations and throw out the nonsensical ones, cleansing the brain of redundant or useless memories.

Others believe that dreams play a different role in information processing. In *Landscapes of the Night,* the late British experimental psychologist and computer scientist Christopher Evans compared the sleeping brain to an off-line computer (one that's not receiving any input from the outside world) that reviews our built-in "programs," the software of daily living, and updates them.

"In every second of every waking hour, there is a veritable bombardment on each of the senses, and the brain is taking in an almighty load of information on thousands of different subjects to add to the body of knowledge it already has," Evans wrote. "During REM sleep—and possibly at other times as well—the brain is scanning this new information, rerunning and rewriting existing programs to see if they are relevant in the light of the day's experience."

Yet something else is also going on. Periodically throughout the night, according to Evans, the mind "eavesdrops" on the brain's work. Our dreams, then, are glimpses of the brain's nightly data processing. Yet that doesn't mean they're insignificant. In ways that scientists can't fully explain, dreams—whatever their psychological content or meaning—serve a very important purpose: They help us work out solutions to a wide variety of daytime problems.

## NIGHT SCHOOL

One of the most fundamental functions of dreams is the learning of new material. Infants spend as much as half their sleep time in REM or dream sleep, perhaps because they have so very much to learn. And we never seem to outgrow our need to "sleep on" new information.

At the University of Ottawa, researchers discovered that students in an intensive language course who learned quickly increased their REM time at night, whereas the slow learners did not. Not surprisingly, those with longer REM periods got better grades. Another experiment studied patients recovering from accidents that had damaged their brains and left them unable to speak, a condition called aphasia. The patients who were making the greatest progress in regaining their speech spent more time in REM than those who weren't improving.

The brain processes more than factual information during the night. Charles Pearlman, M.D., and Ramon Greenberg, M.D., psychiatrists at the Veterans Administration Hospital in Boston, found that patients spent more time dreaming after particularly difficult psychotherapy sessions. In another experiment, volunteers were shown shocking or upsetting movie clips (such as a videotaped autopsy) at two different times. The ones who slept and dreamed before the second screening didn't react as strongly the second time; the ones who'd stayed awake were as upset as they'd been initially, even though they knew what to expect.

# PUTTING YOUR DREAMS TO WORK FOR YOU

Dreaming about your problems is no substitute for facing them head-on during the day. But, says Gayle Delaney, Ph.D., author of *Living Your Dreams,* "Dreams can touch you at a level where you're much less defensive about yourself and your experiences, so you can understand things better." She recommends a technique called dream incubation to harness the wisdom of dreams. Here are the basic steps:

1. At bedtime, record the events of the day in a diary, adding a few brief statements about what's on your mind.
2. Write a one-line phrase that asks the question most pertinent to a problem on your mind, such as "What's going on between us?" or "Why do I always pick friends who are dead ends?"
3. When you turn out the light, repeat the question over and over, like a mantra or lullaby, until you fall asleep.
4. When you wake up, write down whatever comes to mind. Whatever it is, it's relevant.
5. Try, on your own or with a therapist, to match up the echo from the night with a person or situation in your real life.

Dreams may help, not only in assimilating information and experiences but also in preparing for new encounters. British psychologist Nicholas Humphrey, of Cambridge University, has suggested that dreams are "dress rehearsals" for events we anticipate, hope for, or fear in everyday life. In her studies at the University of Cincinatti, Carolyn Winget found that pregnant women who had anxious dreams about labor and delivery, such as losing the baby, giving birth to a monster, or dying in childbirth, had shorter labors than those who'd had more pleasant dreams about giving birth.

But dreams may do more than purge anxiety. In one intriguing experiment, Rosalind Cartwright, Ph.D., chairman and professor of psychology at Chicago's Rush-Presbyterian-Saint Luke's Medical Center, presented student volunteers with realistic problems, such as a situation that triggered sexual guilt or a conflict between work and pleasure. Seven hours later she asked for their suggested solutions.

In the meantime, some of the students stayed awake; others slept in a sleep laboratory—some undisturbed, some only until they entered REM sleep, when they were awakened. The ones who had not slept at all came up with simple Hollywood-style suggestions for the theoretical problems. Those who were allowed to dream without interruption were more likely to deal with the realistic dimensions of the situation.

## NIGHT AND DAY

In real life, the amount of time we spend in REM typically increases during periods of illness, grief, or emotional turmoil—even when we spend less time than usual asleep because of our distress. In a study of women who were particularly prone to irritability and depression because of premenstrual syndrome (PMS), Ernest Hartmann, M.D., director of the sleep laboratory at the Lemuel Shattuck Hospital in Boston, found that while they didn't sleep more than other women, they spent considerably more time dreaming in the nights before their monthly periods.

We all may need to dream more during certain critical times so that we can do what Cartwright calls "emotional reprogramming." As she explains, "When we dream, we reconcile new information to our old self and put it all together so that we can get up and fight another day. Dreams are a way of restoring our sense of competence. When things are going well, we may not need much restoration. After serious problems or disastrous days, it may take more than one night to recoup our losses."

In studies of women going through divorce, Cartwright found that those who were depressed about the end of their marriages entered REM sleep earlier in the night (a characteristic of all depressed patients) and dreamed in the past tense, although they rarely saw themselves as married. The women's dreams clearly reflected their moods and feelings during the day, Cartwright observed. Those who were coping well by day had positive dreams at night; those who were depressed had far less pleasant dreams.

Another prominent dream researcher, Milton Kramer, M.D., director of the Sleep Disorders Center at Cincinnati Hospital in Ohio, sees dreaming as "an emotional thermostat" that helps get us back on an even keel—as he puts it, "back to Go"—by morning. Daytime concerns invariably creep into our nighttime dreams. According to Kramer, young men and women dream more about morality and guilt; the middle-aged, about aggression and sexuality; the elderly, about illness and death. But most dreams are based on the concerns and events of the preceding day.

Two University of Richmond psychologists, Kenneth Blick and Joan Howe, analyzed the dream diaries of twenty-four college women and thirty-seven elderly women. The younger women had more emotions in their dreams, but many were negative, such as anger and fear. A sense of enjoyment and joy accounted for a much higher proportion of the emotions in the dreams of the older women, perhaps reflecting their less stressful, more stable life-style.

In addition to reflecting the past day, dreams may influence the coming day. In his studies, Kramer has found that dreams clearly affect morning moods. Generally, the more people in your dreams, the better you feel the following day. And Kramer believes you can program your dreams to wake up smiling. "It's not that complicated," he says. "Most of us have certain types of dream characters that make us feel good. In my case, it's an older woman—a mother figure, if you will. And so I think about this type of person as I'm falling asleep."

## DIRECTING YOUR DREAMS

Remembering dreams is largely a matter of practice. A nineteenth-century French aristocrat, the Baron d'Hervey, born in 1822, began writing down every dream he could remember when he was in his early teens. During the first six weeks of his journal keeping, he could remember only fragments of dreams. Within six months, he not only recalled complete dreams, but in about a third of the dreams, he realized he was dreaming and consciously directed what was happening—a technique now called lucid dreaming.

With practice, you may be able to do the same. Psychologist Stephen LaBerge, Ph.D., of Stanford University, has developed a method for inducing lucid dreams. Here is a step-by-step guide to the MILD—Mnemonic Induction of Lucid Dreams—process:

1. When you wake in the night, try to focus on the last dream you had, recalling feelings, thoughts, sensations.
2. Spend ten to fifteen minutes reading or doing some-

thing that requires full wakefulness, including something you want to occur in your dreams.

3. Lying in bed, say to yourself: "The next time I dream,
   I want to realize that I'm dreaming."
4. Visualize yourself in bed sleeping. See yourself back in
   your last dream or in another dream, aware that you're
   dreaming.
5. Repeat the last two steps several times.
6. Let yourself fall back to sleep, reminding yourself to
   watch out for feelings that indicate you're dreaming,
   such as anxiety, fear, recurrent themes, or impossible
   situations, such as flying or floating.

Using this approach over a thirty-month period, LaBerge
increased the number of his lucid dreams from four to
twenty a month. To him, lucid dreaming has become a
way to bridge the worlds of waking and dreaming, an
opportunity to explore "new realms of experience."

Once you're aware that you're dreaming, you can rewrite
the scripts of your bad dreams. In one experiment, psychologist Cartwright taught some of the depressed divor-
cées in her research group how to replace their masochistic
dreams with happier plots.

One woman, for example, kept dreaming of walking
along a beach and being swallowed up by a giant wave—
a dream indicating that she was being overwhelmed by
events she couldn't control. Cartwright suggested that the
next time she had this recurring dream, she try swimming.
That's exactly what she did. She imagined herself popping
to the surface and swimming to shore. The nightmare lost
its terror, and she regained confidence in her ability to
cope.

According to a report in the *British Journal of Psychiatry*,
a therapist in Manchester uses a similar approach to help
nightmare sufferers. One seventeen-year-old girl would
wake as often as four times a month because of a terrifying

nightmare that a snake was crawling into her bed. Several times already, she had cut her knee dashing out of bed in fright.

The girl did as the therapist suggested. Every evening she closed her eyes and rehearsed the nightmare. For two weeks, she had no bad dreams, but then the nightmare returned. This time she added a new ending to the dream: She triumphantly cut off the snake's head. Since she still screamed in the night—even though she didn't waken fully—she learned to end the dream even earlier, cutting off the snake's head as soon as it appeared. Soon she was sleeping peacefully through the night.

## BAD DREAMS

Even scary dreams may serve an important function. According to psychologist Jill Morris, author of *The Dream Workbook,* "bad dreams can be catalysts for forcing us to recognize feelings that need our attention, and they can spotlight which of our many emotional needs should have priority at that time."

If you wake from a bad dream, Morris advises asking these questions before trying to return to sleep:

- What am I feeling now?
- How would I like to change my dream?
- What do specific images in the dream remind me of?
- How would I like to deal with the frightening symbols in the dream?

If we consciously explore what's behind our bad dreams, they can become, as Morris puts it, "blessings in disguise. They can give us an invaluable chance to learn to cope with our fear, to experience it fully, instead of running away from it, so that we can handle it better in our waking lives."

Psychiatrist Hartmann, author of *The Nightmare: The Psychology and Biology of Terrifying Dreams,* agrees that our bad dreams can teach us about our strengths and our weaknesses. "Nightmares aren't a horrible influence on the outside trying to get you," he says. "They're a part of you."

While most people have nightmares only once or twice a year, about one person in two hundred has a nightmare every week. According to Hartmann, nightmare sufferers tend to be women who've had a less-than-happy childhood and a difficult adolescence characterized by turmoil, depression, possible drug use, or a suicide attempt. As adults, these women are in fairly good psychological shape but they have "thin boundaries," that is, they don't distinguish clearly between fantasy and reality. This sort of sensitivity makes them more open and vulnerable—traits that may predispose them to artistic expression or to mental illness. Among the creative souls tormented by nightmares were Wagner, Dostoyevski, Hawthorne, Goya, Rimbaud, Poe, Tchaikovsky, and Mark Twain. (See chapter 6 for more information on nightmares.)

Nightmares also can deliver practical messages. One night the man considered one of the founding fathers of modern sleep research, William Dement, M.D., dreamed that he looked at an ominous shadow in his chest X ray and realized that his right lung was infiltrated with cancer. "I will never forget the surprise, joy, and exquisite relief of waking up," he says. He quit smoking immediately.

## CREATIVE DREAMING

Sometimes dreams provide a different form of inspiration. Many writers trace some of their most famous works to dream images. Samuel Taylor Coleridge wrote "Kubla Khan" after a fantastical dream; two classic horror stories—*Frankenstein* and *The Strange Case of Dr. Jekyll and Mr. Hyde*—grew out of the nightmares of Mary Wollstonecraft Shelley and Robert Louis Stevenson. Beethoven and Donizetti based some of their famous melodies on their dreams. Einstein saw the formula, $E = mc^2$, in a dream.

After years of working on a thorny problem, some inventors find the solution in a dream. Elias Howe dreamed that a hostile tribe told him to produce a sewing machine or he would die at the end of a spear. He failed, but the image of the tips of their spears approaching his body gave him the idea of developing a sewing machine with a needle carrying the thread at its tip. After struggling to understand the structure of benzene, the German chemist Friedrich Kekule dreamed of six snakes biting each other's tails in a circle. On waking, he realized that this hexagon represented benzene's molecular structure.

Sometimes dreams, perhaps only by eerie coincidence, seem to foreshadow the future. Abraham Lincoln once dreamed of waking in the night to the sound of sobbing. He wandered through the White House, looking for the source of such anguish. In the East Room he found a crowd of mourners surrounding a casket. Looking into it, he saw his own body and heard someone explain that the president had been slain by an assassin. Within days, the dream became a reality.

The writer Samuel Clemens (Mark Twain) once dreamed that his brother died. In the dream, his brother lay in a metal coffin. On his chest was a bouquet of white flowers with a red blossom in the center. A month later Clemens's brother was killed in an explosion on a Mississippi steamboat. At the funeral, he confronted the same scene he'd seen in his dream, right down to the single red blossom set amid white flowers.

## THE STUFF OF DREAMS

Creative or prophetic dreams are the exception, not the rule. By and large, our dreams are, well, boring. According to thousands of reports from sleepers wakened during REM, dreams tend to be more passive than active, more negative than positive, more unpleasant than pleasant.

From childhood on, men dream more about other men than about women, while women dream equally of men and women. The reason may be that other males are a source of more gratification and more anxiety and stress for men, whereas women find their relationships with both sexes equally pleasurable and equally disturbing. According to Milton Kramer, men's dreams tend to be more active and friendly, yet they're also more likely to include a fight scene. Men also dream more about finding money and appearing naked in public than women do.

For both sexes, dreams usually involve the dreamer and two other persons, and nothing much happens. "Dreaming is really like living," says Milton Kramer, "which also tends to be mundane. When you're talking about your vacation, you don't say that you had two eggs and a small orange juice for breakfast. You describe the highlights. You do the same with your dreams: You forget the dull ones and remember the exciting or scary ones."

Yet even boring dreams, which are just as important as wildly fanciful ones to our brain's nighttime "housekeeping," can be psychologically significant—not because of their content, but because of our interpretation. As an example, Kramer tells of a psychotherapy patient who dreamed of standing between two men. "Now, that sounds boring, but the identities of the two men, the feeling of being torn between them, the relationships that each had with the other, made it fascinating."

Freud believed that all dreams, however mundane, were

significant and argued that trivial dreams held highly disguised messages about the dreamer's unconscious. The newer theories, with their emphasis on the biological aspects of dreaming, suggest that dreams are products of both our bodies and our minds and may have physical as well as psychological significance.

According to this view, a biological reality, such as thirst, might inspire a dream about water. Yet at the same time, what you're doing in the water—whether drowning or swimming, for example—may shed some insight into your psychological state. From this perspective, dreams seem less mysterious, but not necessarily less meaningful. As Milton Kramer emphasizes, "the meaning of a dream always comes externally, not from the dream itself." In other words, only you can decide which dreams are relevant to your waking life and which are nothing more than physiological "noise" in the night.

# CHAPTER 10

# *Getting Help*

*M* ost people know their vital statistics: height, weight, blood pressure, maybe even their cholesterol level or resting heart rate. But they can usually only guess at their nighttime vital signs: how much sleep they need, how long it takes them to fall asleep, how often they wake in the night, how long it takes for them to feel alert in the morning. Yet knowing that information can be critical in identifying and solving a serious sleep problem.

This chapter provides you with self-tests to help you learn more about the way you sleep, as well as advice on where to turn to get help if you need it.

## THE WAY YOU SLEEP

The following questionnaire will reveal the way you *think* you sleep. In answering the questions, reflect back on the nights of the past two weeks and base your answers on your memory of those nights. The questions are designed to help you sort out feelings of sleepiness or alertness as well as the specifics of your daytime and nighttime routine. Many focus on sleep habits, including your nightly sleep schedule, nap times, use of medications, and other behaviors that might affect your sleep.

---

# HOW YOU SLEEP: A SELF-PORTRAIT

1. Are you usually sleepy at bedtime? ☐ Yes, very ☐ Moderately ☐ No, not at all
2. Do you usually follow a sleep ritual before getting into bed? ☐ Yes, always ☐ Usually ☐ Rarely ☐ Never
3. Rate your typical bedtime mood on a scale of 1 to 10:

1    2    3    4    5    6    7    8    9    10
*Anxious*            *Tense*            *Relaxed*

4. What time do you usually go to bed?
5. Is this a regular bedtime? If not, what is your typical weekday bedtime? typical weekend bedtime?
6. How long does it take you to fall asleep on weekdays? on weekends?
7. Do you awaken in the night? How often? How long?
8. What do you do when you wake up in the night or too early in the morning?
9. What time do you usually wake up?
10. What time do you get out of bed on weekdays? on weekends?
11. Rate your typical morning mood on a scale of 1 to 10.

1    2    3    4    5    6    7    8    9    10
*Extremely sleepy*    *Groggy, sluggish*    *Alert, energetic*

12. Do you feel extremely sleepy during the day? Any particular time of day?
13. Do you nap during the day? How often? For how long?

14. How many hours do you typically spend sleeping in a twenty-four-hour period?
15. Are you dissatisfied with how long or how well you sleep?
16. When was the last time you think you slept satisfactorily?
17. Do you use sleeping pills? ☐ Never ☐ Regularly ☐ Occasionally
18. Do you use large amounts of stimulants (coffee, cigarettes, tea, or drugs)?
19. Do you take any medications regularly?
20. What do you think may be the cause of any sleep problems you have?

## BACKGROUND DATA

Only a physician can evaluate your general health and diagnose any specific problems that may be interfering with your sleep. The following questions may make you more aware of symptoms or conditions that could be the underlying cause of a sleep problem. Be sure to bring these to the attention of your doctor or sleep specialist.

### THE STATE OF YOUR BODY
1. Are you generally in good health?
2. Are you overweight? If so, by how much?
3. Do you have any chronic medical problems (high blood pressure, diabetes, or others)?
4. Do you take any medications for these conditions? List name of drug, dosage, and times of administration.
5. When was your last complete physical examination?
6. Were there any unusual findings?
7. List all the major illnesses and injuries of your life, including the dates of onset and recovery times.
8. Have any of these problems led to lingering symptoms? If so, what?

9. Do you have any allergies that you know of? Do you have any symptoms, such as respiratory difficulties, that become worse in different seasons?
10. Do you exercise regularly? How and when?
11. List any health problems, however minor, that you have had in the past three months.
12. List all drugs, prescription and nonprescription, that you have taken in the last month.
13. Is your breathing during the day particularly loud or difficult?
14. Have you ever felt chronically fatigued?
15. Do you feel dizzy or nauseated in the morning but improve during the day?

## THE STATE OF YOUR MIND

Your feelings and thoughts have an enormous impact on your ability to get a good night's sleep. Tension, anxiety, and stress can sabotage your attempts to get to sleep and rest peacefully through the night. The following questions are designed to provide some insight into your emotional life.

1. Have any of the following stressful events occurred to you in the past year: death of spouse, divorce or marital separation, jail term, death of close family member, personal injury or illness, marriage, fired from job, reconciliation with mate after separation, retirement, family illness?
2. Are you a worrier? If so, what do you worry about? Are there certain times when you worry most?
3. Are you impatient?
4. Are you competitive and/or aggressive?
5. Do you get depressed? ☐ Rarely ☐ Occasionally ☐ Often
6. Do you lose interest in other people and things and withdraw into yourself?
7. Do you get angry? ☐ Rarely ☐ Occasionally ☐ Often How do you express your anger?

8. Are you compulsive about your house, work, or studies?
9. Do you take problems from your job home with you? Do you take them to bed with you?
10. Do you tend to ruminate over things that have happened to you?
11. Do you anticipate problems before they arise?
12. How do you respond to pressure?
13. Do you cry? □ Rarely □ Occasionally □ Often How else do you express sadness?
14. Do you have trouble letting go and relaxing?
15. Do you take vacations?
16. Do you confide in people? □ Many people □ A few close friends □ Your spouse □ No one
17. Do you get upset easily? By what?
18. Do you argue with your spouse or other family members? When?
19. Do you believe you acknowledge problems in your life and deal with them directly? Or do you tend to pretend things are going well even when they are not to avoid any conflict?
20. Have you ever seen a psychiatrist or other mental health professional? If so, when? Why? For how long? Why did you stop? Are you currently seeing someone for counseling or therapy? Are you taking any drugs because of a psychiatric problem?

## THE STATE OF YOUR SLEEP ENVIRONMENT

*Where* you lay yourself down to sleep can determine how well you sleep. By asking yourself the following questions, you may be able to pinpoint some common sleep saboteurs, including noise, light, or a worn-out bed. This questionnaire can also help you to identify other behaviors, such as working in bed or frequent traveling, that may be undermining your rest.

1.  How quiet is your bedroom? If it is noisy, what is the source of the noise? What do you do to overcome the noise?
2.  How dark is your bedroom at night and in the morning? Are you ever awakened by the light? Do you ever need to sleep during the day because of your schedule?
3.  Does your bedroom seem too hot or too cold in the night? Do you wake up frequently either to throw off or add a blanket?
4.  Is your mattress comfortable—firm, smooth?
5.  Do you sleep alone?
6.  How big is your bed? Do you feel crowded in it?
7.  What position do you fall asleep in and wake up in?
8.  Have you ever awakened because of your bedmate's snores? movements? kicks?
9.  Do you feel you have a regular sleep-wake schedule? (Verify by comparing against your actual sleep diary.)
10. Do you ever work in bed? How late? How often?
11. What do you do to relax before sleep? Warm bath, music, yoga, breathing exercises, reading, other?
12. Do you ever awaken to care for a child in the night?
13. Do you ever awaken because you are fearful of a prowler or a fire?
14. When was the last time you slept well?
15. What other events in your life coincided with the beginning of your sleep problem?
16. Do you travel often?
17. Do you often shift your work schedule?
18. Do you stay up late or sleep late on certain days of the week?
19. Does anyone in your family have a sleep problem?
20. Ask your bed partner or roommate to describe how you sleep.

## YOUR SLEEP DIARY

To get the most accurate information on your sleep, you need to act as your own "sleep scientist." For the next two weeks, carefully observe your nights and days. Using the forms on pages 194–200, answer the questions in your diary at the appropriate times: your bedtime, when you wake up, or at dinnertime. Keep a clock by your bed so that you can be as accurate as possible in noting when you turn out the light or wake up during the night. These simple facts will help you, or any professionals that you consult, to pinpoint your sleep problems and their probable causes.

## MAKING SENSE OF YOUR SLEEP

After completing the sleep questionnaires and diary, study your answers carefully. If the problem seems to be a straightforward one, such as the fact that you keep irregular hours or chug down coffee late at night, refer back to chapter 2 for information on good sleep habits. If your sleep environment seems to be the culprit, check chapters 2 and 3 for advice. If your problem is falling asleep, chapter 5 provides the latest recommendations on easing your way into sleep. If you can't stay asleep through the night, see chapter 6 for help in overcoming the problems disturbing your rest. If you're sleepy during the day, chapter 7 provides insights into possible reasons why and what to do about them. If you're trying to cope with jet lag, shift work, or a natural tendency toward being a night owl, chapter 8 provides specific recommendations on how to tinker with your biological clock.

If you're unable to figure out what's behind your miserable nights, or if self-help remedies don't work, you should seek professional help. The first person to turn to is your family physician or internist, who will refer you to

a sleep specialist if necessary. Bring the questionnaires in
this chapter with you; your doctor will need much of the
same information in order to evaluate your problem.

A thorough medical workup for a sleep complaint
includes a comprehensive review of both daytime habits
and nighttime rest. Your doctor will want information on
many subjects, including the following:

- The nature, history, and duration of your complaint
- Your past sleep history, including any problems
- Medical history, including head injuries, neurological
  disorders, impotence
- Past and present psychiatric symptoms, diagnoses, and
  treatments
- Use of prescription and nonprescription medications:
  sleeping pills, stimulants, nose drops, pain relievers,
  antihistamines, diet pills, and so on
- Use of caffeine, alcohol, cigarettes, or "recreational"
  drugs
- A detailed description of your sleep habits, environment,
  partner, napping, use of alarm clocks or other waking-
  up aids, exposure to light and dark, bedtime and wake-
  up rituals, when you go to bed and get up, how long
  before you fall asleep, duration of sleep, awakenings,
  how satisfied you are with your sleep, your feelings
  about sleep, what you think about when in bed, your
  expectations about sleep
- Evidence of unusual behavior during sleep: snoring,
  shortness of breath, gasping, breathlessness, bed-
  wetting, sleepwalking, falls in the night, night terrors,
  nightmares, thrashing about in bed, unusual movements,
  leg jerks or cramps, morning headaches, difficulty awakening, sleep paralysis, vivid hallucinations on waking,
  dreams
- Timing of sleep: when you go to bed, whether you nap
  voluntarily or involuntarily, any tendency to be a morning lark or a night owl

- Daytime abnormalities, such as excessive sleepiness, dozing, fatigue, muscle weakness
- A social and occupational history, including your daily habits, job hours, exercise, diet
- Family history of medical and psychiatric conditions, sleep patterns, excessive sleepiness, sleep disorders

Your doctor may get additional information from the following:

- A complete physical examination, with special attention to problems in the upper airway, enlarged tonsils or adenoids, large tongue, short neck, malocclusion of the jaws, obesity
- Analysis of two weeks of your sleep diary, including bedtimes, wake-up times, amount of time needed to fall asleep, duration of sleep, number and duration of awakenings, early-morning wakenings, naps, involuntary sleepiness during the day, use of sleeping pills, coffee, alcohol, stimulants
- Interview with your bed partner
- A tape recording of the sounds you make while sleeping (if indicated because of snoring or other unusual behavior)

## TYPES OF SLEEP PROBLEMS

Diagnosing a sleep disorder can be a complex process because the ailments that disturb our rest are as varied as those that perturb our days. The official classification of sleep disturbances lists more than 120 distinct problems, which are organized into the following categorics:

- Disorders of Initiating and Maintaining Sleep (DIMS), or the insomnias. These include transient insomnia, which is common in healthy, normal people at times of stress, as well as chronic insomnia, which can be caused by psychiatric problems, alcoholism and drug abuse, medical conditions, pain, apnea, abnormal movements during sleep, or environmental factors.

- Disorders of Excessive Sleepiness (DOES). These are characterized by inappropriate sleep without obvious reason. Two major causes are sleep apnea and narcolepsy.
- Disorders of the Sleep-Wake Cycle. These include sleep complaints associated with jet lag, shift work, and de-layed-sleep syndrome.
- The Parasomnias, or abnormal behaviors during sleep. These include bed-wetting, sleepwalking, night terrors, nocturnal asthma, and epilepsy.

The chart below identifies the symptoms of the major sleep disorders.

---

## THE SIGNS OF THE MAJOR SLEEP DISORDERS

### DISORDERS OF INITIATING AND MAINTAINING SLEEP

| | |
|---|---|
| Transient Insomnia | Triggered by a specific stress<br>Less total sleep time<br>Longer time to fall asleep<br>Lasts for less than three weeks |
| Chronic Insomnia | Slightly increased time to fall asleep<br>Essentially normal total sleep time<br>Self-perception that there has been less sleep time than has actually occurred<br>Better sleep in unfamiliar surroundings<br>Sleep does not feel refreshing |

| Depression (Major) | Decreased total sleep time |
| | Decreased time before REM begins |
| | Less deep non-REM sleep |
| | Early-morning awakening |
| | Symptoms of depression: loss of energy, appetite, sexual desire; problems concentrating; sadness; and so on |
| Depression (Bipolar or Manic) | Increased total sleep time |
| | Excessive sleepiness |
| | Feelings of sadness |
| Anxiety | Increased time to fall asleep |
| | Decreased time asleep |
| Psychosis or Mania | Increased time to fall asleep |
| | Decreased time asleep |
| | Acute symptoms of psychosis (hallucinations, delusions, and so on) |
| **Use of Depressant Drugs** | |
| Tolerance | Less deep sleep |
| | Less REM |
| | More light non-REM sleep |
| | Fragmented sleep |
| Withdrawal | Less total sleep |
| | More intense REM sleep and vivid nightmares |
| | More awakenings |
| | Nausea, cramping |
| **Use of Stimulant Drugs** | |
| Tolerance | Increased time to fall asleep |
| | Less total sleep |
| | Less deep sleep |
| | Less REM |
| | Anxiety |
| | Irrationality |
| | Paranoid thinking |

| | |
|---|---|
| Withdrawal | Increased total sleep time<br>Less time to fall asleep<br>Daytime sleepiness<br>Depressed mood |
| Use of Alcohol<br>  Tolerance | Less REM sleep<br>Increased awakenings in second half of night |
| Acute<br>withdrawal | Longer time to fall asleep<br>More REM sleep<br>Increased movements during sleep<br>Irritability |
| Long-term<br>changes | More light stage-1 non-REM sleep<br>Less deep stage-4 non-REM sleep<br>Increased wakefulness |
| REM-<br>Interruption<br>Insomnia | Multiple awakenings during dreaming |

## DISORDERS OF EXCESSIVE SLEEPINESS

| | |
|---|---|
| Sleep Apnea | At least thirty partial arousals during the night because of breath stoppages lasting ten seconds or longer<br>Snoring<br>Feeling of unrefreshing sleep<br>Daytime fatigue<br>Headaches<br>Night sweats<br>Choking<br>Less deep non-REM sleep (Stages 3–4)<br>More light non-REM sleep (Stages 1–2) |
| Leg<br>Movements<br>(Nocturnal<br>Myoclonus) | Repeated leg contractions lasting five to ten seconds and occurring in at least three groupings of thirty movements each, lasting minutes |

| | |
|---|---|
| Restless Legs | Feelings of not sleeping or unrefreshing sleep<br>Signs of "tearing up" the bed while asleep<br>Daytime fatigue<br>Irresistible urge to move legs when sitting or lying down<br>Association with neurological diseases |
| Narcolepsy | Irresistible daytime sleepiness<br>Attacks of muscle weakness<br>Feeling of paralysis upon awakening<br>Vivid, frightening hallucinations when waking<br>REM periods begin within ten minutes of falling asleep |
| Sleep Drunkenness | Grogginess upon awakening<br>Increased amounts of deep non-REM sleep<br>Falling back to sleep, if given the chance, in morning |

## PARASOMNIAS

| | |
|---|---|
| Sleepwalking | Complex movements, including sitting, standing, or walking, in the first third of the night |
| Night terrors | Greatest incidence during first third of the night<br>Increased heart rate<br>Rapid breathing<br>Confusion and agitation for five to ten minutes after waking from an attack |
| Bed-wetting | Children may be confused, disoriented, and hard to arouse after an episode |

| Nightmares | Awakening from dream |
| | Lack of confusion |
| | Anxiety |
| | Ability to recall dream |
| Teeth Grinding (Bruxism) | Rhythmic movement of jaws |
| | Increased movements of arms and legs |

Ultimately you and your doctor will decide whether or not you should be evaluated at a sleep center. If your sleep problem is interfering with the way you feel and function during the day, you may need the special expertise only such centers can offer.

## WHAT TO EXPECT AT A SLEEP CENTER

Sleep medicine is one of the newest medical specialties. Two decades ago there were only a few special facilities for people with sleep problems. Now there are more than one hundred clinical sleep disorders centers in the United States, where experts in a variety of fields—psychiatry; neurology; respiratory medicine; urology; and ear, nose, and throat surgery—work together to unravel and solve sleep problems.

Sometimes your sleep history alone—for example, years of waking up screaming in the night—will pinpoint exactly what the problem is (night terrors, in this case). If your primary complaint is excessive daytime sleepiness, you might undergo a daytime procedure called a Multiple Sleep Latency Test. At two-hour intervals throughout the day, you will be hooked up to a polysomnograph—a machine that monitors brain waves, heart rhythm, respiration, and other bodily functions—and allowed to nap.

For other sleep complaints, you may have to undergo an all-night sleep evaluation.

This test, unlike most medical procedures, involves no injections, no anesthetics, no incisions, no X rays, and no discomfort other than the slight initial irritation of the electrodes attached to your face and scalp. All you have to do is sleep. If you're afraid that you won't be able to sleep in an unfamiliar setting, be assured that many others have felt the same way. Sleep specialists can recognize and discount most "first-nighter" effects.

You will come to the sleep center in the late evening, several hours before your usual bedtime. Your bedroom will be comfortable and quiet, with an intercom so that you can speak to a technician at any time in the night. You can bring your own pajamas, pillow, and nighttime reading material.

Once you're ready for bed, technicians will attach several electrodes to your face and body. These are placed *on* the skin, usually over an ointment dabbed on the skin to form a better seal. All are arranged in pairs, so that if one falls off during the night, the other will serve as a backup. While they don't hurt, the electrodes may feel irritating at first, like insects that have landed on your face.

Two electrodes are placed on the chin to record muscle tension; two, at the corner of the eyes to measure eye movements; two, on the scalp to detect brain waves. Other electrodes on the upper right and lower left of the chest measure heartbeats. One on each leg records movements. A temperature-sensitive device may be taped under your nostrils and at your mouth to record breath rate and volume of inhaled air. A beltlike gadget around the lower chest monitors the movements of your diaphragm.

The electrodes will be hooked up to the central line of the polysomnograph equipment. Although the wires are firmly secured, they are not confining. You will be able to sit up, turn to either side, and, usually with the technician's help in "unplugging" yourself, get up and go to the bathroom.

The technician will make note of when you turn out the light and, by watching the brain waves recorded on the polysomnogram, when you fall asleep. All night long the electrodes will send signals to the polysomnograph; these are converted into electrical impulses that appear as wavy lines on continuous sheets of paper. In the course of a single night, squiggles and waves will cover half a mile of paper.

In the morning, you will be asked questions about how you slept, including estimates of how long it took for you to fall asleep, how often you awakened, and how this night compared with a normal night's sleep. With the aid of a computer, a trained polysomnographer will assess the data recorded from your sleeping body and brain. Some centers may ask you to spend an additional night in order to supply further information.

The costs of an all-night sleep evaluation vary, but two nights of polysomnography and a complete analysis of your sleep patterns can run as much as one thousand dollars. Medicare, Medicaid, and many insurance companies cover such fees, but you should always check your policy.

**FINDING A SLEEP CENTER**

Most major medical centers, particularly those affiliated with medical schools, have some physicians with expertise in sleep medicine on their staff. You can check with the departments of psychiatry or neurology.

The Association of Sleep Disorders Centers, which accredits specialized sleep clinics, has provided the following list of centers in the United States and abroad:

*ASSOCIATION OF SLEEP DISORDERS CENTERS*
*Accredited Members*


## Alabama

Sleep Disorders Center of Alabama
Affiliated with Baptist Medical Center Montclair
800 Montclair Road
Birmingham, Alabama 35213
Attn: Vernon Pegram, Ph.D.
205-592-5650

Sleep/Wake Disorders Center
University of Alabama
University Station
Birmingham, Alabama 35294
Attn: Drs. Wooten and Faught
205-934-7110

Sleep Disorders Center
The Children's Hospital of Alabama
1600 Seventh Avenue South
Birmingham, Alabama 35233
Attn: Drs. Wooten and Lyrene
205-939-9386


## Arizona

Sleep Disorders Center
Good Samaritan Medical Center
1111 East McDowell Road
Phoenix, Arizona 85006
Attn: Richard M. Riedy, M.D.
602-239-5815

Sleep Disorders Center
University of Arizona
1501 North Campbell Avenue
Tucson, Arizona 85724
Attn: Stuart F. Quan, M.D.
602-626-6112

**Arkansas**

Sleep Disorders Diagnostic and Research Center
University of Arkansas for Medical Sciences
4301 West Markham, Slot 555
Little Rock, Arkansas 72205
Attn: Drs. Scrima and Hiller
501-661-5528

**California**

WMCA Sleep Disorders Center
Western Medical Center—Anaheim
1025 South Anaheim Boulevard
Anaheim, California 92805
Attn: Louis McNabb, M.D.
714-491-1159

Sleep Disorders Center
Scripps Clinic and Research Foundation
10666 North Torrey Pines Road
La Jolla, California 92037
Attn: Richard M. Timms, M.D.
619-455-8087

UCLA Sleep Disorders Clinic
Department of Neurology
710 Westwood Plaza, Room 1184 RNRC
Los Angeles, California 90024
Attn: Emery Zimmermann, M.D., Ph.D.
213-206-8005

Sleep Disorders Center
Holy Cross Hospital
15031 Rinaldi Street
Mission Hills, California 91345
Attn: Elliott R. Phillips, M.D.
818-898-4639

Sleep Disorders Center
U.C. Irvine Medical Center
101 City Drive South
Orange, California 92668
Attn: Jon Sassin, M.D.
714-634-5777

Sleep Disorders Center
Sequoia Hospital
Whipple and Alameda
Redwood City, California 94062
Attn: Drs. Votteri and Pavy
415-367-5620

Sleep Disorders Clinic and Research Center
Saint Mary's Hospital
450 Stanyan Street
San Francisco, California 94117
Attn: Donald Nevins, M.D.
415-750-5579

Sleep Disorders Program
Hoover Pavilion, 2nd Floor
Stanford University Medical Center
Stanford, California 94305
Attn: German Nino-Murcia, M.D.
415-497-6601

Sleep Disorders Center
Torrance Memorial Hospital
3330 Lomita Boulevard
Torrance, California 90509
Attn: Lawrence W. Kneisley, M.D.
213-235-9110, x2049

**Colorado**

Sleep Disorders Center
Presbyterian Medical Center
1719 East 19th Avenue
Denver, Colorado 80218
Attn: Ian Happer, M.D.
303-839-6447

Sleep Disorders Center
University of Colorado Health Sciences Center
700 Delaware Street
Denver, Colorado 80204
Attn: Drs. Reite and Zimmerman
303-592-7278

## Connecticut

Sleep Disorders Center
The Griffin Hospital
130 Division Street
Derby, Connecticut 06418
Attn: Drs. Sewitch and Liebmann
203-735-7421, x560

New Haven Sleep Disorders Center
100 York Street
Suite 2G
New Haven, Connecticut 06511
Attn: Drs. Watson and Sholomskas
203-776-9578

## Florida

Sleep Disorders Center
Mount Sinai Medical Center
4300 Alton Road
Miami Beach, Florida 33140
Attn: Martin A. Cohn, M.D.
305-674-2613

## Georgia

Sleep Disorders Center
Northside Hospital
1000 Johnson Ferry Road
Atlanta, Georgia 30342
Attn: James J. Wellman, M.D.
404-851-8135

**Hawaii**

Sleep Disorders Center
Straub Clinic and Hospital
888 South King Street
Honolulu, Hawaii 96813
Attn: James W. Pearce, M.D.
808-523-2311, x8448

**Illinois**

Sleep Disorders Center
University of Chicago
5841 South Maryland, Box 425
Chicago, Illinois 60637
Attn: Jean-Paul Spire, M.D.
312-962-1780

Sleep Disorders Center
Rush-Presbyterian-Saint Luke's
1753 West Congress Parkway
Chicago, Illinois 60612
Attn: Rosalind Cartwright, Ph.D.
312-942-5440

Sleep Disorders Center
Methodist Medical Center of Illinois
221 N.E. Glen Oak
Peoria, Illinois 61636
Attn: Drs. Morgan and Lee
309-672-4966

## Kentucky

Sleep Disorders Center
Humana Hospital Audubon
One Audubon Plaza Drive
Louisville, Kentucky 40217
Attn: Carl P. Browman, Ph.D.
502-636-7459

## Louisiana

Tulane Sleep Disorders Center
Department of Psychiatry and Neurology
1415 Tulane Avenue
New Orleans, Louisiana 70112
Attn: Gregory Ferriss, M.D.
504-587-7457

## Maryland

The Johns Hopkins University Sleep Disorders Center
Francis Scott Key Medical Center
Baltimore, Maryland 21224
Attn: Philip L. Smith, M.D.
301-955-0571

National Capital Sleep Center
4520 East West Highway, Number 406
Bethesda, Maryland 20814
Attn: Wallace B. Mendelson, M.D.
301-656-9515

## Michigan

Sleep Disorders Center
Henry Ford Hospital
2799 West Grand Boulevard
Detroit, Michigan 48202
Attn: Frank Zorick, M.D.
313-972-1800

## Minnesota

Sleep Disorders Center
Methodist Hospital
6500 Excelsior Boulevard
Minneapolis, Minnesota 55426
Attn: Mark K. Wedel, M.D.
612-932-6083

Sleep Disorders Center
Neurology Department
Hennepin County Medical Center
Minneapolis, Minnesota 55415
Attn: Mark Mahowald, M.D.
612-347-6288

Sleep Disorders Center
Mayo Clinic
200 First Street SW
Rochester, Minnesota 55905
Attn: Philip R. Westbrook, M.D.
507-285-4150

## Missouri

Sleep Disorders Center
Saint Louis University Medical Center
1221 South Grand Boulevard
St. Louis, Missouri 63104
Attn: Kristyna M. Hartse, Ph.D.
314-577-8705

Sleep Disorders Center
Deaconess Hospital
6150 Oakland Avenue
St. Louis, Missouri 63139
Attn: James K. Walsh, Ph.D.
314-768-3100

**New Hampshire**

Sleep Disorders Center
Department of Psychiatry
Dartmouth Medical School
Hanover, New Hampshire 03756
Attn: Michael Sateia, M.D.
603-646-7534

**New York**

Sleep-Wake Disorders Center
Montefiore Hospital
111 East 210th Street
Bronx, New York 10467
Attn: Michael J. Thorpy, M.D.
212-920-4841

Sleep Disorders Center
Columbia Presbyterian Medical Center
161 Fort Washington Avenue
New York, New York 10032
Attn: Neil B. Kavey, M.D.
212-305-1860

Sleep Disorders Center
Saint Mary's Hospital
89 Genesee Street
Rochester, New York 14611
Attn: Donald W. Greenblatt, M.D.
716-464-3391

Sleep Disorders Center
Department of Psychiatry
SUNY at Stony Brook
Stony Brook, New York 11794
Attn: Theodore L. Baker, Ph.D.
516-444-2916

Sleep-Wake Disorders Center
New York Hospital–Cornell Medical Center
21 Bloomingdale Road
White Plains, New York 10605
Attn: Charles Pollak, M.D.
914-997-5751

**Ohio**

Sleep Disorders Center
Mercy Hospital of Hamilton/Fairfield
1275 East Kemper Road
Cincinnati, Ohio 45246
Attn: Martin B. Scharf, Ph.D.
513-671-3101

Sleep Disorders Center
Department of Neurology
Cleveland Clinic
Cleveland, Ohio 44106
Attn: Dudley S. Dinner, M.D.
216-444-8732

Sleep Disorders Evaluation Center
Department of Psychiatry
Ohio State University
Columbus, Ohio 43210
Attn: Helmut S. Schmidt, M.D.
614-421-8296

## Oklahoma

Sleep Disorders Center
Presbyterian Hospital
N.E. 13th at Lincoln Boulevard
Oklahoma City, Oklahoma 73104
Attn: William Orr, Ph.D.
405-271-6312

## Oregon

Sleep Disorders Program
Good Samaritan Hospital
2222 N.W. Lovejoy Street
Portland, Oregon 97210
Attn: Gerald B. Rich, M.D.
503-229-8311

## Pennsylvania

Sleep Disorders Center
Jefferson Medical Center
1015 Walnut Street, Third Floor
Philadelphia, Pennsylvania 19107
Attn: Karl Doghramji, M.D.
215-928-6175

Sleep Disorders Center
The Medical College of Pennsylvania
3300 Henry Avenue
Philadelphia, Pennsylvania 19129
Attn: June M. Fry, Ph.D., M.D.
215-842-4250

Sleep Disorders Center
Western Psychiatric Institute
3811 O'Hara Street
Pittsburgh, Pennsylvania 15213-2593
Attn: Charles F. Reynolds III, M.D.
412-624-2246

Sleep Disorders Center
Department of Neurology
Crozer-Chester Medical Center
Upland-Chester, Pennsylvania 19013
Attn: Calvin Stafford, M.D.
215-447-2689

**Tennessee**

BMH Sleep Disorders Center
Baptist Memorial Hospital
899 Madison Avenue
Memphis, Tennessee 38146
Attn: Helio Lemmi, M.D.
901-522-5704

Sleep Disorders Center
Saint Thomas Hospital
Post Office Box 380
Nashville, Tennessee 37202
Attn: J. Brevard Haynes, Jr., M.D.
615-386-2068

**Texas**

Sleep-Wake Disorders Center
Presbyterian Hospital
8200 Walnut Hill Lane
Dallas, Texas 75231
Attn: Howard P. Roffwarg, M.D.
214-696-8563

Sleep Disorders Center
All Saints Episcopal Hospital
1400 Eighth Avenue
Fort Worth, Texas 76104
Attn: Edgar Lucas, Ph.D.
817-927-6120

Sleep Disorders Center
Department of Psychiatry
Baylor College of Medicine
Houston, Texas 77030
Attn: Ismet Karacan, M.D.
713-799-4886

Sleep Disorders Center
Humana Hospital Metropolitan
1303 McCullough
San Antonio, Texas 78212
Attn: Sabri Derman, M.D.
512-223-4050

Sleep Disorders Center
Scott and White Clinic
2401 South 31st Street
Temple, Texas 76508
Attn: Francisco Perez-Guerra, M.D.
817-774-2554

**Utah**

Intermountain Sleep Disorders Center
LDS Hospital
325 Eighth Avenue
Salt Lake City, Utah 84143
Attn: Drs. Walker and Farney
801-321-3417

## Wisconsin

Sleep Disorders Center
Gundersen Clinic, Ltd.
1836 South Avenue
La Crosse, Wisconsin 54601
Attn: Martin L. Engman, M.D.
608-782-7300

*PROVISIONAL MEMBERS*
*(June 1986)*

## Alabama

Sleep Disorders Lab
Carraway Methodist Medical Center
1600 Twenty-Sixth Street North
Birmingham, Alabama 35234
Attn: Richard M. Champion, M.D., F.C.C.P.
205-226-6164

SAMC Sleep Disorders Center
Post Office Drawer 6987
Dothan, Alabama 36302
Attn: Drs. Prince and Watson
205-793-8134

North Alabama Sleep Disorders Center
Huntsville Hospital
101 Sivley Road
Huntsville, Alabama 35801
Attn: Paul Legrand, M.D.
205-533-8020

**Arkansas**

Sleep Disorders Center
Baptist Medical Center
9601 I-630, Exit 7
Little Rock, Arkansas 72205-7299
Attn: Drs. Galbraith and Phillips
501-227-4750

**California**

Sleep Disorders Institute
Saint Jude Hospital and Rehabilitation Center
101 East Valencia Mesa Drive
Fullerton, California 92634
Attn: Drs. Roethe, Sturman, and Petrie
714-871-3280

Loma Linda Sleep Disorders Center
Loma Linda University Medical Center
11234 Anderson Street
Loma Linda, California 92354
Attn: Michael Bonnet, Ph.D.
714-825-7084, x2703

Sleep Disorders Center
Hollywood Presbyterian Medical Center
1300 North Vermont Street
Los Angeles, California 90027
Attn: Drs. McGinty and Rothfeld
213-660-3530

Sleep Disorders Center
The Hospital of the Good Samaritan
616 South Witmer Street
Los Angeles, California 90017
Attn: F. Grant Buckle, M.D.
213-977-2206

Sleep Disorders Center
Pomona Valley Community Hospital
1798 North Garey Avenue
Pomona, California 91767
Attn: Drs. Zinke, Desai, Nicholson, and Kack
714-623-8715, x2135

Sleep Disorders Center
San Jose Hospital
675 East Santa Clara Street
San Jose, California 95112
Attn: Drs. Choslovsky and Connor
408-977-4445

Sleep Disorders Center
South Coast Medical Center
31872 Coast Highway
South Laguna, California 92677
Attn: Drs. Pittluck and deBerry
714-499-1311, x2186

## Colorado

Porter Regional Sleep Disorders Center
Porter Memorial Hospital
2525 South Downing
Denver, Colorado 80210
Attn: Richard Mountain, M.D.
303-778-5723

## District of Columbia

Sleep Disorders Center
Georgetown University Hospital
3800 Reservoir Road N.W.
Washington, D.C. 20007
Attn: Samuel J. Potolicchio, Jr., M.D.
202-625-2697, x2020

## Florida

Sleep Disorders Center
Sacred Heart Hospital
5151 North 9th Avenue
Pensacola, Florida 32504
Attn: Frank V. Messina, M.D.
904-476-7851, x4128

## Idaho

Idaho Sleep Disorders Center
Saint Luke's Regional Medical Center
190 East Bannock
Boise, Idaho 83712
Attn: Bruce T. Adornato, M.D.
208-386-2440

## Illinois

Sleep Disorders Center
Neurology Service
Veterans Hospital
Hines, Illinois 60141
Attn: Meenal Mamdani, M.D.
312-343-7200, x2326

Sleep Disorders Clinic and Laboratory
Carle Clinic and Hospitals
611 West Park Street
Urbana, Illinois 61801
Attn: Drs. Picchietti and Greeley
217-337-3364

## Indiana

Sleep Disorders Center
Saint Mary's Medical Center
3700 Washington Avenue
Evansville, Indiana 47750
Attn: David Howard, M.D.
812-479-4257

Regional Sleep Studies Laboratory
The Lutheran Hospital of Fort Wayne, Inc.
3024 Fairfield Avenue
Fort Wayne, Indiana 46807
Attn: Bruce J. Hopen, M.D.
219-458-2001

Sleep Disorders Center
Winona Memorial Hospital
3232 North Meridian Street
Indianapolis, Indiana 46208
Attn: Frederick A. Tolle, M.D.
317-927-2100

Sleep Disorders Center
Lafayette Home Hospital
2400 South Street
Lafayette, Indiana 47903
Attn: Fredrick Robinson, M.D.
317-447-6811

## Iowa

Sleep Disorders Center
Iowa Methodist Medical Center
1200 Pleasant Street
Des Moines, Iowa 50308
Attn: Randall R. Hanson, M.D.
515-283-6207

Sleep Disorders Center
Department of Neurology
University of Iowa Hospitals and Clinics
Iowa City, Iowa 52242
Attn: Quentin Stokes Dickens, M.D.
319-356-2571

## Kansas

Sleep Disorders Center
Wesley Medical Center
550 North Hillside
Wichita, Kansas 67214
Attn: Arnold M. Barnett, MRCP, FACP
316-688-2660

## Kentucky

Sleep Disorders Center
Saint Joseph's Hospital
1 Saint Joseph Drive
Lexington, Kentucky 40504
Attn: Robert Granacher, Jr., M.D.
606-278-3436

Sleep Disorders Center
Good Samaritan Hospital
310 South Limestone
Lexington, Kentucky 40508
Attn: George W. Privett, Jr., M.D.
606-278-0352

## Louisiana

Sleep Disorders Center
Touro Infirmary
1401 Foucher
New Orleans, Louisiana 70115
Attn: Gihan Kader, M.D.
504-891-7087

Sleep Disorders Center
Willis-Knighton Medical Center
2600 Greenwood Road
Shreveport, Louisiana 71103
Attn: Nabil A. Moufarrej, M.D.
318-632-4823

## Massachusetts

Sleep Disorders Center
Boston University Medical Center
75 East Newton Street
Boston, Massachusetts 02146
Attn: George F. Howard III, M.D.
617-247-5206

Sleep Disorders Center
Boston Children's Hospital
300 Longwood Avenue
Boston, Massachusetts 02115
Attn: Richard Ferber, M.D.
617-735-6242

Sleep Disorders Unit
Harvard University School of Medicine
Beth Israel
330 Brookline Avenue
Boston, Massachusetts 02215
Attn: Drs. Jean Matheson and J. Woodrow Weiss
617-735-3237

Sleep-Wake Disorders Unit
University of Massachusetts
55 Lake Avenue North
Worcester, Massachusetts 01605
Attn: Sandra Horowitz, M.D.
617-856-3802

## Maryland

Maryland Sleep Diagnostic Center
Ruxton Towers, Suite 211
8415 Bellona Avenue
Baltimore, Maryland 21204
Attn: Thomas E. Hobbins, M.D.
301-494-9773

## Michigan

Sleep Disorders Clinic
Catherine McAuley Health Center
Post Office Box 995
Ann Arbor, Michigan 48106
Attn: William T. Allen, M.D.
313-572-3093

Sleep Disorders Center
University of Michigan Medical Center
1405 East Ann Street
Ann Arbor, Michigan 48109
Attn: Michael S. Aldrich, M.D.
313-763-5118

Sleep Disorders Center
Ingham Medical Center
401 West Greenlawn Avenue
Lansing, Michigan 48909
Attn: Paul Gouin, M.D.
517-374-2510

## Minnesota

Sleep Disorders Center
Fairview Southdale Hospital
6401 France Avenue South
Edina, Minnesota 55435
Attn: Drs. Corson and Zarling
612-924-5058

## Mississippi

Sleep Disorders Center
Division of Somnology
University of Mississippi
Jackson, Mississippi 39216
Attn: Lawrence S. Schoen, Ph.D.
601-987-5552

## Missouri

Sleep Disorders Center
Research Medical Center
2316 East Meyer Boulevard
Kansas City, Missouri 64132-1199
Attn: Ronald Chisholm, Ph.D.
816-276-4222

Sleep Disorders Center
Saint Mary's Hospital
101 Memorial Drive
Kansas City, Missouri 64108
Attn: Iftekhar Ahmed, M.D.
816-756-2651

## North Carolina

Sleep Disorders Center
Charlotte Memorial Hospital
Post Office Box 32861
Charlotte, North Carolina 28232
Attn: Dennis Hill, M.D.
704-331-2121

Sleep Disorders Center
Division of Neurology
Duke University Medical Center
Durham, North Carolina 27710
Attn: Rodney Radtke, M.D.
919-681-3344

## Nebraska

Sleep Disorders Center
Lutheran Medical Center
515 South 26th Street
Omaha, Nebraska 68103
Attn: Drs. Ellingson and Roehrs
402-536-6352

## New Hampshire

Sleep-Wake Disorders Center
Hampstead Hospital
East Road
Hampstead, New Hampshire 03841
Attn: J. Gila Lindsley, Ph.D.
603-329-5311, x240

**New York**

Sleep Disorders Center
Winthrop-University Hospital
259 First Street
Mineola, New York 11501
Attn: Alan M. Fein, M.D.
516-663-2005

**North Dakota**

TNI Sleep Disorders Center
Saint Luke's Hospital
5th Street at Mills Avenue
Fargo, North Dakota 58102
Attn: Philip M. Becker, M.D.
701-280-5673

**Ohio**

Sleep/Wake Disorders Laboratory
Miami Valley Hospital Suite G200
Thirty Apple Street
Dayton, Ohio 45409
Attn: Martin B. Scharf, Ph.D.
513-220-2515

Sleep Disorders Center
Bethesda Oak Hospital
619 Oak Street
Cincinnati, Ohio 45206
Attn: Milton Kramer, M.D.
513-569-6320

Northwest Ohio Sleep Disorders Center
The Toledo Hospital
2142 North Cove Boulevard
Toledo, Ohio 43606
Attn: Frank O. Horton III, M.D.
419-471-5629

## Oklahoma

Sleep Disorders Center
Saint Francis Hospital
6161 South Yale
Tulsa, Oklahoma 74136
Attn: Richard M. Bregman, M.D.
918-494-1350

## South Carolina

Sleep Disorders Center
Baptist Medical Center
Taylor at Marion Streets
Columbia, South Carolina 29220
Attn: Drs. Bogan and Ellis
803-771-5557

## Tennessee

Sleep Disorders Center
Saint Mary's Medical Center
Oak Hill Avenue
Knoxville, Tennessee 37917
Attn: Michael L. Eisenstadt, M.D.
615-971-6011

Sleep Disorders Center
Fort Sanders Regional Medical Center
1901 West Clinch Avenue
Knoxville, Tennessee 37916
Attn: Ronald W. Bryan, M.D.
615-971-1375

**Texas**

Sleep Disorders Center
Sun Towers Hospital
1801 North Oregon
El Paso, Texas 79902
Attn: Gonzalo Diaz, M.D.
915-532-6281

Sleep Disorders Center
Sam Houston Memorial Hospital
1624 Pech
Post Office Box 55130
Houston, Texas 77055
Attn: Todd Swick, M.D.
713-468-4311

Sleep Disorders Center
Pasadena Bayshore Medical Center
4000 Spencer Highway
Pasadena, Texas 71504
Attn: Drs. Bradley and Stein
713-944-6666

**Utah**

Sleep Disorders Center
Utah Neurological Clinic
1055 North 300 West, Suite 400
Provo, Utah 84604
Attn: John M. Andrews, M.D.
801-379-7400

## Virginia

Sleep Disorders Center
Norfolk General Hospital
600 Gresham Drive
Norfolk, Virginia 23507
Attn: Reuben H. McBrayer, M.D.
804-628-3322

Sleep Disorders Center
Community Hospital of Roanoke Valley
Post Office Box 12946
Roanoke, Virginia 24029
Attn: Thomas W. DeBeck, M.D.
703-985-8435

## Washington

Sleep Disorders Center
Providence Medical Center
500 Seventeenth Avenue, C-34008
Seattle, Washington 98124
Attn: Ralph A. Pascualy, M.D.
206-326-5366

## Wisconsin

Sleep Disorders Center
Columbia Hospital
2025 East Newport Avenue
Milwaukee, Wisconsin 53211
Attn: Paul A. Nausieda, M.D.
414-961-4650

Sleep Disorders Center
Milwaukee Children's Hospital
1700 West Wisconsin Avenue
Milwaukee, Wisconsin 53201
Attn: Thomas B. Rice, M.D.
414-931-4016

## ACCREDITED LABORATORIES FOR SLEEP-RELATED BREATHING DISORDERS

### California

Sleep Apnea Center
Merritt-Peralta Medical Center
450 Thirtieth Street
Oakland, California 94609
Attn: Drs. Kram and Nusser
415-451-4900, x2273

Southern California Sleep Apnea Center
Lombard Medical Group
2230 Lynn Road
Thousand Oaks, California 91360
Attn: Ronald A. Popper, M.D.
805-495-1066

### New Jersey

Sleep Disorders Center
Newark Beth Israel Medical Center
201 Lyons Avenue
Newark, New Jersey 07112
Attn: Monroe S. Karetzky, M.D.
201-926-7597

### Pennsylvania

Sleep Disorders Center
Mercy Hospital of Johnstown
1127 Franklin Street
Johnstown, Pennsylvania 15905
Attn: Drs. Hanzel and Parcinski
814-533-1000

## GOOD NIGHT, AMERICA!

This book began with a bedtime story of a desperate quest for sleep. It ends with a very different tale:

Once again, it's time for bed. You look back briefly on a full day. Despite your busy schedule, you made time for regular tension time-outs and for a long walk in the early evening. You had your last cup of coffee at lunch and your last sip of alcohol with dinner. Half an hour ago, you put aside your work notes and household chores and began the slow, sweet process of getting ready for bed with some soft music, a soothing bath, a quiet chat with your spouse, a few gentle stretches.

As you slide between the sheets, you repeat a familiar litany in your mind: "I'm so sleepy. The bed feels so wonderful. I'll be asleep in seconds." Most nights the next thing you know, the alarm is buzzing, and a new day awaits. You wake feeling refreshed and ready for anything.

This book provides all you need to know to rewrite your own bedtime story. By following its advice and recommendations, you can assure yourself of a happy ending—for all the days and the nights of your life.

# YOUR SLEEP DIARY BEDTIME LOG

|  | Day 1 | Day 2 | Day 3 | Day 4 |
|---|---|---|---|---|
| Date: | | | | |
| Sleepiness, on a scale of 1 to 10:<br>1  2  3  4  5  6  7  8  9  10<br>*Alert*    *Drowsy*    *Extremely tired* | | | | |
| Mood, on a scale of 1 to 10:<br>1  2  3  4  5  6  7  8  9  10<br>*Anxious*    *Tense*    *Relaxed* | | | | |
| Describe activities from dinner until bedtime. | | | | |
| Presleep ritual: describe each step up to getting into bed. | | | | |
| What was the actual time you got into bed? | | | | |
| Describe activities before lights-out. | | | | |

194

| | Day 5 | Day 6 | Day 7 | Day 8 |
|---|---|---|---|---|
| Did you take a sleeping pill? If so, write down name and amount. | | | | |
| Have you had any alcohol in the past four hours? If so, write down what and how much you drank. | | | | |
| How much coffee have you had today? in the last six hours? | | | | |
| How many cigarettes have you smoked today? in the last six hours? | | | | |
| What time did you eat dinner? | | | | |

# YOUR SLEEP DIARY BEDTIME LOG

| | Day 5 | Day 6 | Day 7 | Day 8 |
|---|---|---|---|---|
| Date: | | | | |
| What have you eaten since dinner? | | | | |
| Have you used any drugs (prescription or nonprescription) today? List specific drugs and amount used. | | | | |
| Have you had any physical problems or discomfort during the day? If so, describe. | | | | |
| Have you had any unusually stressful experiences today? Have you felt particularly relaxed, uptight, sad, or elated? | | | | |
| Did you exercise during the day? Indicate what you did and when. | | | | |
| Sum up your thoughts and feelings about your day. | | | | |

## YOUR SLEEP DIARY WAKE-UP LOG

| | Day 9 | Day 10 | Day 11 | Day 12 |
|---|---|---|---|---|
| Estimate the time you fell asleep last night. | | | | |
| Did you wake up in the night? How often? How long did you stay awake each time? | | | | |
| What did you do when you awakened in the night? | | | | |
| What time did you wake up in the morning? | | | | |

197

# YOUR SLEEP DIARY WAKE-UP LOG

| | Day 9 | Day 10 | Day 11 | Day 12 |
|---|---|---|---|---|
| Did you wake up before or after the alarm? | | | | |
| What time did you get out of bed? | | | | |
| Indicate how well you slept on a scale of 1 to 10:<br>1 2 3 4 5 6 7 8 9 10<br>*Very poorly*    *Very well* | | | | |
| Indicate your energy level on a scale of 1 to 10:<br>1 2 3 4 5 6 7 8 9 10<br>*Very tired*    *Groggy*    *Refreshed, energetic* | | | | |
| Estimate your total sleep time during the night. | | | | |

# YOUR SLEEP DIARY DINNERTIME LOG

| | Day 13 | Day 14 | Day 15 | Day 16 |
|---|---|---|---|---|
| Were you extremely sleepy during the morning or during the afternoon? | | | | |
| Did you take any naps? When? For how long? | | | | |
| How much time did you sleep during the day? | | | | |
| Estimate how much time you have slept in the past twenty-four hours. | | | | |

# YOUR SLEEP DIARY DINNERTIME LOG

| | Day 13 | Day 14 | Day 15 | Day 16 |
|---|---|---|---|---|
| Describe your functioning (creativity, concentration, decision making, and so on) in the morning and in the afternoon on a scale of 1 to 10:<br><br>1  2  3  4  5  6  7  8  9  10<br>*Inadequate   Adequate   Peak, outstanding* | | | | |
| Using the same scale, describe your feelings and ability to cope in the morning and in the afternoon. | | | | |
| Describe your emotions during the day. | | | | |
| Describe your physical state during the day. | | | | |

# Index

# *About the Author*

Dianne Halcs is a nationally known expert on sleep. She is national spokesperson for the Better Sleep Council, a nonprofit organization that promotes public awareness of the importance of sleep to good health. Author of *The Complete Book of Sleep* and co-author of *The U.S. Army Total Fitness Program*, Ms. Hale has also written for *Parade, The New York Times, Woman's Day, Mademoiselle,* and *American Health.*